FRANCESCA SEGAL

Mother Ship

VINTAGE

This book is about my own personal experience, and that of my daughters. With the exception of my family, a few close friends and their children, most names here have been changed, together with identifying personal details. Hospitals are and should be places of privacy for patients and staff alike, and I have therefore done my best to preserve the anonymity of the people whose stories intersected with my own.

1 3 5 7 9 10 8 6 4 2

Vintage
20 Vauxhall Bridge Road,
London SW1V 2SA

Vintage is part of the Penguin Random House group of companies whose addresses can be found at global.penguinrandomhouse.com

 | Penguin
Random House
UK

First published in Vintage in 2020
First published in hardback by Chatto & Windus in 2019

penguin.co.uk/vintage

A CIP catalogue record for this book is available from the British Library

ISBN 9781784709464

Printed and bound in Great Britain by Clays Ltd, Elcograf S.p.A.

Quote on p.205 from 'Days' by Philip Larkin

Penguin Random House is committed to a sustainable future for our business, our readers and our planet. This book is made from Forest Stewardship Council® certified paper.

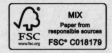

For A-lette and B-lette

Generations of women have asserted their courage on behalf of their own children and men, then on behalf of strangers, and finally for themselves.

Adrienne Rich, *Of Woman Born*

PREFACE

DAY MINUS ONE

Thursday, 1st October

Identical girls felt like a lottery win.

For the first time in my life I was part of a posse; I was a one-woman girl gang. Pregnancy was like performing a perpetual magic trick, to move around the world in the silent company of my daughters. Two tiny sidekicks always there, shifting just below the hot, taut skin. I was writing a novel. Together we sought out the sunniest desks in the library and there spent long afternoons, some of us reading, others napping. We shared a new and urgent interest in anchovies, and cottage cheese. On Tuesdays and Thursdays, the three of us did Pilates. At night I dreamed them into being, but during the day I didn't have to for I felt them – they were there and with me, wild for sugar, protesting little pugilists if I had the temerity to drink iced water. At my fortnightly visits to the hospital Multiples Clinic the sonographers would tut a bit, fussing that both babies were measuring small, but before my eyes they wheeled and flipped with great energy, and they were growing, steadily. Everything was as it should be. At every midwife appointment I received rave reviews for blood pressure, for blood sugar, for appropriately substantial weight gain, for being a sensibly mainstream blood group. Despite being over the age of thirty-five and carrying twins, my pregnancy was plain sailing. I felt excellent. I have not surveyed my friends widely, but I believe I was probably smug, and unbearable.

And so it was with shock that I sat up in bed one morning, twenty-nine weeks and six days' pregnant, to discover that I'd wet myself. I wondered if there was some way I might whip the sheet from under Gabe as he slept on beside me, as a circus clown pulls a tablecloth from beneath a china tea set. Maybe he would never have to know? But when I reached for my phone to google 'sudden pregnancy incontinence', the screen's white glow revealed that what had begun to leak from me was blood.

Most of the next thirty-six hours were dull. At the Central Hospital I was put on an antenatal ward and told that I needed to stay in for twenty-four hours' observation; each 'episode' would reset the clock. Six, eight hours would pass, I would be given permission to dress and venture out for some air, I would bleed again, and then be rushed to the labour ward where nothing would happen, and then I would be back up on antenatal in a room of women, variously crying. I was not crying, because, unlike them, I was not in the throes of having a baby. I had ten more weeks, a full quarter of a pregnancy ahead. On my last scan Baby A had measured somewhere around two pounds, Baby B was smaller. The weight of four packets of butter, or a few apples. Less than a bag of sugar. They couldn't come now, I remember thinking, and so they wouldn't. I was very calm.

Around midnight I shambled to the loo, closing myself into the bathroom with relief at the brief solitude, at the relative silence. But suddenly it came again, and this time within seconds much of the floor was slick with blood; I left a trail of vivid footprints as I backed towards the sink. Still, I couldn't seem to take on board that this was Not Good;

I mostly felt bad for the hospital cleaners. When it seemed to have stopped I used the convenient handrails to heave myself down on to all fours and, with a wad of remarkably unabsorbent aquamarine paper towels, I began to mop up the floor. It was from this position, on hands and knees, my breathing heavy with effort, that the emergency cord caught my attention. Its bright red toggle seemed for some reason to resonate. *How clever it is*, I thought, from my position on the smeared tile, *that someone could reach that cord even from down here*. My own face confronted me at the unexpected bottom of a full-length hospital mirror, chalk-white. Then, almost as a passing thought, *You should maybe think about pulling it*.

When the nurse arrived I was full of reflexive apologies for the disturbance, for the mess. By now, still kneeling, much of the blood was soaking its way up my trailing hospital gown. The nurse did not seem to find it cute when I said I was tidying up. *Leave that*, she snapped. *Come*.

What did I think, then, padding obediently behind her, back down to the labour ward for the final time? I can barely remember, but I believe that those were, at thirty-five, my last, belated hours of a Peter Pan childhood. It now seems impossible, but even then, I was still convinced it would all turn out all right. It had been a long day and Gabe had only gone home to sleep an hour earlier; I wanted him beside me, but I didn't want him to be tired. I didn't call.

Downstairs I was trussed up with the sort of straps one might use to move a wardrobe, which held in place two Dopplers to monitor Twin 1 and Twin 2, and a third monitor, measuring the contractions I was not yet having. Tiny, galloping hoof beats; a herd of miniature wild horses thundering across a miniature plain. Everyone on the inside was still all right. So it seemed it was me who was bleeding, inconveniently, insistently.

I phoned Gabe around 6 a.m. and caught him already up and dressed, about to come back to the hospital. If not this then for what, exactly, would I bother him, he wanted to know? He arrived, irritable with me, but bearing breakfast, nonetheless. I looked at it with longing. While he was downstairs buying me a pot of lava-hot porridge, it had been decided that I should be nil by mouth just in case. *Just in case I need a C-section*, I told him wildly, as though I had found myself among incompetents, among lunatics who must nonetheless be humoured. *Isn't that insane?*

I remained hungry the rest of the day, until around 3 p.m. when my accumulated uneventful hours won me a reprieve. Gabe went foraging, and returned with two sandwiches. I ate both his and mine. Chicken and avocado, oozing mayonnaise, and a second course of cheddar and sliced tomato on generously buttered brown bread. Then I had a cinnamon Danish pastry and half of Gabe's blueberry muffin. As we ate, we talked. Though I hadn't known it, at midnight while I was cleaning the hospital floor, my daughters had passed across a magical threshold, from twenty-nine weeks to thirty, at which statistics change, outcomes improve. Two-pound babies have uncertain futures. Respiratory distress syndrome from immature lungs. Irreversible lung damage from long-term ventilator support. Pneumonia. Brain bleeds. Cerebral palsy. Anaemia. Retinopathy of Prematurity, which can cause partial or total blindness. Sepsis. Necrotising Enterocolitis – life-threatening bowel death. I knew none of these words then, but I understood that if we could buy my daughters another week, another two, another five, their prognosis would be materially different. And now they were not twenty-nine weeks but thirty. For the next few months I would take it easy – I could write, after all, in bed.

I ate, and ate. I drank a litre of water. Then I stood up sated, relieved, and a blood clot like a piece of calves' liver slithered from me to the floor. The doctor was bleeped, and returned to tell me that I had run out of chances.

The anaesthetist will be in soon, and I'm going to ask someone from the NICU to come up and talk to you. His eyes passed over the sandwich boxes, the muffin papers, the crumbs down the straining front of my hospital gown. *Try not to vomit on my operating table*, he advised as he left.

The theatre was busy and so we had maybe half an hour to come to terms with what was now happening, to me, to Gabe, to Babies A and B. We used most of it to take photos of Gabe in his hospital scrubs and to giggle like overtired schoolchildren, fuddled by a narcotic combination of ignorance and spectacular denial. *Why put off till December what you can do today?* I cried, and wondered aloud if this meant I had really got away with a twin pregnancy and no stretch marks. A midwife came with a cartoonishly large pair of scissors, to cut from my wrist a series of neon cotton friendship bracelets, grubby survivors of a visit to a hippy market on a summer holiday to Ibiza. I was surprised to find that some quiet, unobtrusive part of myself must have taken this episode seriously when I realised I had already removed my earrings and wedding ring before leaving home. No one knew we were here, no parents, no siblings, no friends, and that increased the feeling of truancy from meaningful reality. Then a new doctor appeared in the doorway, fair-haired and serious, with a soft Swedish accent and a careful bedside manner that recalled me to the reality that we were at a hospital bedside. She introduced herself – a registrar on the Neonatal Intensive Care Unit. She was so kind to us, and her kindness was sobering. *I wanted to explain to you what will happen to your daughters after the birth.* Our giggles subsided. It was some time, after that, before we laughed again.

MOTHER SHIP

DAY ZERO

Friday, 2nd October

2/10/15 – P. Miller (midwife)

16.10 Preparing for anaesthetic CSE [combined spinal &
epidural anaesthesia]

16.37 Operation commenced – Cat. 3 EMCS

16.39 Twin 1 delivered – given to Neonatal team

16.41 Twin 2 delivered – given to Neonatal team

16.43 Placenta delivered – ragged, incomplete and in
poor condition. Obstetrician aware. Sent to histology.

17.24 Operation complete. Estimated Blood Loss ~~400ml~~ 500ml

17.34 Transferred to theatre bed, washed and dried

The midwife's notes then draw the episode to a brief close, stating simply:

17.40 Plan: Recover

She made it sound so easy.

*

I didn't meet my daughters the day that they were born. After surgery I lay in the recovery bay in the honeyed fog of diamorphine until I was wheeled to a single room. How grateful I was to be shielded from the jolly chaos and high feeling of the adjacent ward, with its bawling and balloons, where other women who had recently given birth had babies beside them: huge, tight-swaddled, hard-won trophies shown off to troops of admiring visitors, their birth stories now behind them. The ward was shielded from me, too. No one in the ecstatic flush of fresh motherhood should have to glimpse an empty bedside. The street name for diamorphine is heroin, and with gratitude I gave myself up into its arms.

I don't know how long I slept before Melanie came; a pixie midwife with a glittering blue stud in her nose and a 1ml syringe in her hand not much bigger than a pencil lead. Did I think, she asked, we might just try expressing? They will soon need colostrum downstairs, in Neonatal Intensive Care.

I was cranked to semi-vertical and Melanie showed me, earnest student of a torturously painful manoeuvre called something like the C-shaped clamp and squeeze. The two of us worked doggedly together, clamping, squeezing, but my breasts had expected another several months before their work commenced, and they were as unprepared as the rest of me. I had the vague thought that circulating heroin in my bloodstream might not be ideal for the babies to ingest; in the end I lay back on the pillow to regard the ceiling, leaving Melanie to her kneading and pummelling. I winced as silently as I could. Eventually she departed with a triumphant 0.4mls – eight drops. Still nil by mouth, this will apparently be enough to keep them both going, whenever they are ready. When she left I began, for the first time, to cry. Taking my unready daughters from within me felt not like a birth but an evisceration. They were elsewhere and in need of me, and needing more than I could give them. To stem the tears I closed my eyes, just for a moment, and awoke the following morning.

DAY ONE

Saturday, 3rd October

Though it is 4 a.m. I feel clear as a bell, able to stand, to walk, to request the removal of the catheter that I will otherwise, God help me, remove myself. Last night I was drugged; this morning I am electrified. Somewhere in this hospital are my daughters.

I make my way down the corridor to the lift, grateful to my surgeon that I can walk, slow and stately, but incontestably erect. Twelve hours have passed since my Caesarean section. I have put in my contact lenses, after the irrational but I suppose factually correct thought that my babies have never seen me in glasses. For our reunion I would like to look like myself.

Neonatal Intensive Care Unit. The doors of the NICU are always locked and at this hour there is no one on reception. I stand outside for a long time, rocking from foot to foot to ease the tightening vice of backache of which I am only now becoming aware, for all the world as if I am trying to soothe a baby. Finally a passing doctor spots me and buzzes me in. Do I know where I'm going? I shake my head, no. What kind of a mother doesn't know where to find her children? It seems I am sobbing; how odd I hadn't noticed until now. She shows me to some sinks and I wash my hands. *I think the new twins are this way*, she says, and I think, *My daughters*.

At this hospital the Neonatal Intensive Care Unit has wards of four beds, and a minimum of two nurses present on each ward at all times, two babies assigned to each nurse. The soundtrack is a combination of control tower, server room and a busy canteen, as orders are called out, and a thousand toaster ovens ping, over and over. It is dark but for the banks of monitors, displaying incomprehensible data. It could be the cockpit of a space ship.

Each small astronaut has a temperature monitor, an oxygen saturation probe, a series of heart monitors, and most have TPN, Total Parenteral Nutrition, a mix of glucose, protein and lipids provided by an intravenous pump. Any and all of these machines can beep, either to alert the nurses to a problem or sometimes simply just to say a quick *hello, no problem at present.* The babies in this room, Room One, are not well babies: one or other of their alarms go off somewhere in the region of once a minute, sometimes continuously.

Over time, I will come to find the five rising notes of the TPN infusion pump particularly appalling, for this usually indicates that an intravenous cannula has been dislodged or occluded and another one will need to be inserted, another procedure, another vein punctured. Beeping of any sort will set me on edge for a long time: at home I will develop a habit of standing vigil by the microwave to stop it just before it finishes.

These two on the left, side by side in two incubators, these two, says the doctor, they are my daughters. The room is in shadows, and each lies in a pool of sapphire light, for jaundice. A is doll-sized; B is smaller still. Their skin is too fragile for clothes. They have been positioned on their stomachs, curled in deep oval nests of rolled towels and rough hospital sheets printed with faded clowns beneath A, faded teddy bears beneath B. They are both wearing white cloth hats, white Velcro sunglasses, and their noses and mouths are obscured by a mask delivering Continuous Positive Airway Pressure, CPAP, to force their stiff, unready lungs to breathe. A feeding tube disappears between their lips and down their throats. Their faces remain a secret known only to each other.

They have no fingernails, no toenails, and later when they lose the Audrey Hepburn shades I will see they have no brows or lashes. These are not essential components of a human being for my daughters are clearly humanoid, or perhaps superhuman in their appearance. I press my face to the glass. I see red starfish hands, and fleshless arms, bone-shaped. I can trace their circulation, the fine leaf-veining of tributaries clearly visible beneath their backs' translucent skin. The exquisite transgression of their forming selves exposed, caught in the act of becoming. I feel my intrusion upon them: they were not ready.

They are the furthest from me, and the furthest from one another that they have ever been. I do not recognise them. They are otherworldly in their strangeness, and oceanic in their beauty. They are half-beings in the half-light and in an instant my heart shatters, and I become half a mother, twice.

*

After another fruitless session with a midwife and a syringe, I return to the NICU where I am formally introduced to the maniacal hygiene protocol: bags and all outer garments in lockers in the hallway – it's better, if you can, to keep a full change of clothes here, ones that haven't been contaminated by exposure to the real world beyond these walls, to the Tube or the bus or even the hallways. No wristwatches or bracelets. No long nails, false nails, no rings with gems or crevices. Absolutely no long sleeves. At the entrance to the ward is a series of sinks and I am taught to turn off taps with my elbows, dripping hands raised as if I am scrubbing up for surgery, to dry them thoroughly on abrasive disposable towels and finally to massage them with several pumps of stinging alcohol gel. To reach my children in Nursery One I must then walk ten paces straight ahead and turn left where, having shouldered my way through a single swing door and touched nothing, the hand-washing and alcohol gel ritual must be repeated. It is an obsessive-compulsive's paradise, here. One cannot be too fastidious: wiping a single tear from your cheek is enough to transmit an infection. One great fear is Respiratory Syncytial Virus, RSV. A healthy adult experiences RSV as a mild cold, but in a premature infant it can turn very quickly into deadly bronchiolitis or pneumonia. We are at the beginning of the RSV season, which runs the same time as that other October-to-March killer, the flu. There are thirty-three babies here, thirty-three immune systems in various stages of immaturity and compromise. To enter is a responsibility.

Then the nurse shows me to a small space, not much larger than a closet, and immediately beside the lockers: the expressing room, which I have already learned, from eavesdropping, to call the milking shed.

The milking shed is an innocuous enough space for what is, incontestably, the central seat of power on the unit. Mothers here must express milk eight to ten times every twenty-four hours, and each session can take up to forty minutes. If my milk ever comes in, I will spend a lot of time in here.

There are eight chairs and four breast pumps, a sink for more hand washing, a cardboard box of endlessly replenished disposable pumping paraphernalia, and a large number of supportive leaflets. I am grateful for these leaflets, and will study them without irony.

In addition there are posters lobbying for skin-to-skin 'Kangaroo Care', for breastfeeding long into toddlerhood, and further posters advising us what to do if our husbands are abusive. There is a curling sheet of paper stuck beside the taps, reminding us of the proper procedure for washing hands. The two prime positions are side by side at the back, facing the wall, where a small shelf serves as a table, somewhere to rest a drink and a magazine. Everyone else must sit in a circle behind these seats, trapped into sociability by the ergonomics of the room. It is like being in a military helicopter, pilot and co-pilot at the front, and everyone else in a close ring behind.

The milking shed is not a place of modesty. This is a place of exposure, of lifted hijabs, of dropped veils and dropped pretences. Walking in for the first time is unnerving, like approaching the table of popular girls at school lunch. It feels as if everyone knows one another and one another's case histories. Here lie unknown alliances and factions.

But I will soon learn that it is quite unlike school, and entirely unlike cliques I've known before, and feared. There is kindness in this room. There is generosity of spirit and a sharing of wisdom. Which doctors know the most, which have a fearsome bedside manner, which nurses most faithfully record desats and bradys (as I will learn to call their drops in blood oxygen, their drops in heart rate). Which nurses will always make time to help you have (the always uppercase) Cuddles. What time the daily ward round takes place in each nursery; when the sonographer is likely to be coming round to do the brain scans; which nearby beauty salon can quickly remove the nail extensions you applied for a party last week before accidentally giving birth on your friend's bathroom floor thereby, ironically, missing the party. I am not a user of such words nor am I a feeler of such feelings, but the milking shed is a place, a state, of grace. Today I sit down silently in a room of strangers, expressing and expressing. I have no milk. But women talk here while their own bottles fill, and I listen at their feet like a disciple.

*

Our twins populate the left half of Nursery One. In Bed Three is William, whose parents were there when I went down this morning, busy with tasks I cannot imagine. In Bed Four is Martin. I met his mother, Sunny, in the hallway, as I was coming back up here. Sunny is here with her own mother, who speaks only Korean and whose name I will never know, though I will come to be fond of her. She is petite and short-haired, self-effacing, manifestly religious. She has flown from Busan to pray by the cotside and to stand in for Martin's father, who works long shifts.

When I can no longer tolerate the discomfort of standing uselessly between the incubators, I return to my own bed upstairs. It becomes clear that I have, as I was earlier warned not to do, 'overdone it'. I try to sleep, but I am relentlessly accosted by kindly midwives who take my blood pressure and administer medication. Most also have designs on my breasts. Today, my children are nourished by an intravenous solution of glucose and lipids, A's through her left wrist, B's through her right, but they cannot expect such special treatment to go on for ever. Tomorrow they will have to try digesting, like the rest of us.

Gabe brings chicken soup: apparently bone broths are good after blood loss. As we eat lunch, we discuss the girls' ward mates, both of whom have names, William and Martin, while our children remain Twin One and Twin Two. We must get to it, but for now it seems so unimportant, compared with the business of keeping them alive. We hadn't even made a shortlist.

Martin is, we decide, a wonderfully optimistic choice. Martin surely will thrive, will one day grow to contented middle-age to fulfil the destiny of his birth certificate. William evokes a freckle-faced Just William, marauding with his Outlaws, cherished piebald mouse in his pocket. But we have only glimpsed William and Martin from afar, and in stealthy peripheral vision. The room is big, and the expanse of empty floor between our incubators is impassable. I quickly intuit that it isn't done to look at other babies, nor at their ministering parents. I do not yet minister. All I have done so far is stand around. Then someone brought me a stool, so for variety I sat on it.

*

When I stagger back down to the NICU after my chicken soup, the mother from Bed Three, William's mother, is washing her hands beside me. She is neat-waisted and slender, and there is no sign that she has recently been pregnant. There are several such women here – either their pregnancies did not extend enough to make substantial alteration to their bodies, or their children have been resident here so many months that they long ago shed their baby weight. This woman's dark hair is long and straight and very shiny, falling to hide her face. Today she is in a blue dress, and scuffed brown pixie boots. She looks young, and worried. Her battered leather phone case is gilded and decorated, like a Bible, and on this basis alone I presume she is a religious Christian. When we've passed on the ward she has, thus far, not met my eye.

I introduce myself. I am buoyant with adrenalin, with shock, with drugs. Sophie, it turns out, is an old-timer, subdued by weeks of relentless anxiety. I am jarring. I say everything wrong. We exchange our vital statistics – the gestational age of our children, and their birth weights. It's how I imagine prisoners might meet one another – crime and time. Sophie's son William was twenty-eight weeks and had severe intra-uterine growth restriction. He was born in August; it is now October and he is still in Intensive Care. At birth he was six hundred grams. *Oh, sweet*, I say. I have not yet learned to talk here. I have not yet understood. *Well, no*, Sophie says, shortly. *It isn't*. She pumps alcohol gel on her hands and leaves, and I listen to the swift clip-clip of her boots as she hurries back to her son's bedside. I wait a moment, to give her time to finish at the next sinks.

Very soon, Sophie will become one of the most treasured women in my life. She will spur me on like a sergeant. She will lift me up like an angel. She will make me laugh with shocking black humour and shameless smut, like a messmate. Sophie saw my daughters before I did, she remembers their arrival: the doctors' fight to stabilise them. She heard their first, thin cries. Sophie was my birth partner, though I didn't know it. Today, however, she is a stranger whom I have affronted, faintly hostile, and with whom I will now have to coexist.

Sophie also writes. A long time later, when I read her version of our first meeting it is eye-opening, which is to say it is unrecognisable to me. In it she praises my erect posture immediately after abdominal surgery, going on to note that unlike many women I refused a wheelchair for my first visits to the NICU, instead walking down myself. That much is true. Her account was written with the myopia of loving hindsight but still, to be ambulant was the most for which she could praise me, then. I know that I offended her, though she claims not to remember. Later I think I exhausted her into being my friend. I was everywhere – on the ward, in the milking shed – and in the end she simply stopped resisting.

DAY TWO

Sunday, 4th October

I thought I'd be the only person in the milking shed at 6 a.m. but like an all-night diner it never closes, merely waxes and wanes in popularity. So this morning I met Lisa, a tiny blonde who grinned and said, *I think I saw your husband naked yesterday.* Apparently Gabe forgot to lock the bathroom when he was changing into his street clothes last night and in a hurry Lisa threw the door open and exposed him to the busy locker room. I doubt anyone batted an eyelid; there is such an accelerated intimacy here. While this conversation takes place, Lisa and I are ourselves both topless, after all.

It turns out that Lisa grew up near me and, though we have never met before, we have several friends in common. Lisa's daughter Emma had intra-uterine growth restriction and Lisa suffered pre-eclampsia, which made for a pregnancy mostly spent pacing the halls of her local hospital with a raging headache, wild with boredom. When the doctors said she would have to deliver Emma at thirty-one weeks, Lisa announced she was popping home to get her washbag and instead came straight here, the Central Hospital, a Level Three unit capable of handling even the most complex or baroque neonatal complications. Compared to my girls, Lisa's little Emma is quite grown up; she was born ten days ago.

I tell her I keep waiting for a doctor to make an overture, to introduce themselves as our daughters' physician, to sit us down behind a consultant's broad leather-topped desk to explain – perhaps with diagrams and drawings – what has and will happen. One has to intercept them to find out anything at all, but to flag down a medic here is like trying to hail a Formula One racing car as a taxi.

You need to catch them on ward round, Lisa explains. Apparently all the doctors come round as a pack each morning visiting each incubator in turn, briefing the nurses in charge, making decisions for the day's care. For parents, ward round offers the crucial five minutes in which to pose any questions they have accumulated over the past twenty-four hours. *And then if there's anything you don't understand,* Lisa says, *write it down and bring it to the milking shed. There's always someone here who knows the answers.*

So today, thanks to Lisa, Gabe and I are ready and waiting for ward round. The consultant arrives, freshly unboxed from his shelf at central casting, a grey-haired man in a burgundy button-down shirt and pale chinos, followed by a gallery tour group of others, some in mufti, most in scrubs. No one is introduced. They could be junior doctors, medical students, pharmacists, dieticians, paediatric aerobics instructors or campaigning local politicians, for all I know. My own name is an equal irrelevance – both in the second and third person I am merely *Mum.*

Twin One is sleeping after a troubled, unstable night. She is manifestly not enjoying what she's seen of the world so far. Breathing is tiring. Her lungs are stiff. She cannot settle and overnight was wasting precious energy, awake and in distress. The consultant rattles open the portholes of her incubator to feel her fontanelle, check her colour, palpate her abdomen. His touch is confident, and untender. His hands are obscenely large around her; her limbs smaller than his thick fingers. The baby does not appreciate the examination, and protests by sounding every alarm at her disposal – her heart is racing; her oxygen levels plummet. The nurse reaches up to silence the bells, and the consultant continues. We await his verdict like a judge's sentence.

I arrange my features into those of someone who understands. One of the junior doctors is writing at speed while the consultant addresses them, nodding intermittently. It occurs to me that it might not be very mature to pretend to comprehend what in fact I do not, when life-altering decisions are being made. But my children do not appear to require mothering. Instead they need sophisticated medical intervention, and I have it in mind that I will somehow be expected to provide it, if I want to be allowed to keep them. I fear that exposing my bewilderment will summon social services. *Not up to it,* the junior doctor might be writing at this moment (while sitting on my stool, I might add), *she didn't know what the TPN was for, let alone how to deal with the bilirubin situation.*

It takes self-confidence to say, *I don't know* and, *Can you tell me?* As they talk, a fogged half-comprehension clarifies into something solid, a single sentence, like water frozen instantly to ice: *I am unable to care for my children.* I remain expressionless, listening.

Someone else continues with her list of medications. I'm fairly sure I heard something that sounded like caffeine but surely could not have been. Something else was 'deranged' (I don't think it was the baby's mother, though you never know). She's pink, which is good, even though she's also yellow, which is bad. Intercostal sounds like it has something to do with the beach. A something in her brain is dilated, but we are not to worry, or at least not until a repeat neurological ultrasound tomorrow when we will be told whether we ought in fact to worry a great deal.

This discussion ends abruptly, with everyone clear on how they are proceeding, though from my perspective it might have been a conversation in Akkadian. The group makes their way from Cot 1 to Cot 2. There is some off-duty chatting amongst themselves, in between. As they reconvene I shuffle over and Gabe and I take up identical sentry posts, beside our other daughter. It feels faintly comical, like an episode of *Fawlty Towers* in which the concierge becomes a waiter by stepping two feet to the left and changing hats. But there is nothing comical about the searing pain that has begun to grip my lower back. As they begin a similar introduction – Twin Two Female Infant Segal, born at thirty plus zero, 1.175kg – my knees almost buckle with it. I grip the side of the incubator and Gabe moves to bring me a chair, but I will not sit down and gaze up like a child at a group of adults, talking to one another over my head. I rock on the balls of my feet. I gather that Twin Two – Baby B, to use our own more intimate nickname for her – is being flooded with antibiotics to fight suspected sepsis, but that on the up side, she is now having a single millilitre of breast milk an hour direct into her stomach, to supplement the intravenous nutrients that run through her leg. This is a major development – her inaugural attempt at digestion. Sepsis sounds extremely not great. But I understand so little that I cannot even formulate a question beyond, *Are they going to be okay?*

The consultant replies with averages, with statistics, with outcomes, with contingents. *We can't make any promises*, he says, and I sense that he might be losing his patience with these women, day after day, demanding of him clairvoyance. Not only is he meant to rescue our children but he is meant to explain in layman's terms precisely how he is doing it, to an endless parade of damp and sagging women in wheelchairs, in gowns, in shock, patients themselves but not (thankfully) his patients. I stand a little straighter, grateful that I fought my way into my maternity jeans and I am not, at least, here in pyjamas. My head is filled with an electric buzz of pain.

When they move on we must leave the room – you are not allowed to hear anyone else's ward round. With one hand on the wall I make my way back to my locker, where I have stashed the codeine. I am repeating *dilated bilateral horns (B)* and *ventricular asymmetry (A)* over and over, in order to remember. Gabe is already on his phone, consulting Dr Google. I plan to collapse in the expressing room, and ask whoever is in there just what the hell is going on inside my children's brains. *Dilated bilateral horns. Ventricular asymmetry. Sepsis.* Already I've learned that the answers are not likely to be found on the ward, but in the milking shed.

*

I cannot lounge around upstairs in bed like a maharani and hand-express colostrum for ever, not least because soon, probably tomorrow, I will be discharged from hospital and will no longer have a wipe-clean plastic bed upstairs on which to lounge. Without continuous medical intervention my two-pound children cannot regulate their body temp-eratures, nor take in calories, nor can they breathe.

So when I go home tomorrow they will not, I am told, be coming. Other hospitals in other countries make provisions for the parents of very premature babies to remain with them twenty-four hours a day, taking charge of as much of their care as is practicable, but though the Central Hospital NICU is new, there is no such provision here. I have taken charge of nothing but the battlefield of my own resistant breasts. I am nominally the mother of two children but I have not held a baby, nor changed a nappy nor, beneath their hats and masks and white felt goggles, have I seen my daughters' eyes or noses or heads. I do not know if they have hair, nor what colour it might be if they do. When the nurse needs it to write notes, I don't even have a stool to sit on near their incubators. In order to stand I take Nurofen and Co-codamol, at permitted intervals.

The consultant would not be drawn on prognoses or outcomes. It is too early, and the road ahead of them is a long one and reliably unpredictable. So we have only averages to go on, and the roiling poisonous vat of Google search results. Chance of cognitive impairment, of physical impairment, of survival. Their chances of suffering a brain bleed are high, but Lisa told me in the milking shed that if we can only make it to seventy-two hours without such a catastrophe the risk of it will fall, and we will have crossed another small but significant threshold.

In the UK, 60,000 babies are born prematurely each year. Of these, most (85 per cent) are classified 'moderate to late preterm', born between thirty-two and thirty-seven weeks; 11 per cent are considered 'very preterm', born between twenty-eight and thirty-two weeks, and the remainder, the 'extremely premature', born before twenty-eight weeks. At thirty weeks on the nose, we sit squarely in the middle of the 'very preterm' box. Whatever might lie ahead, it is becoming clear that my children's stay in hospital is at present indefinite while mine will be a modest three days. Tomorrow I must return to sleep at home, where everything and nothing will be the same.

DAY THREE

Monday, 5th October

Parents whose infants are well enough to be held (for what is universally known as 'Cuddle Time') must change into clean hospital gowns, worn backwards so that they open at the front to permit skin-to-skin contact. Kangaroo Care – prolonged periods of skin-to-skin with a parent – has been shown to stabilise a premature baby's heart, respiration and temperature, which in turn fattens them up by preventing the expenditure of unnecessary calories. A lactating mother's breasts have been shown to change temperature according to the needs of the infant they hold; supposedly while holding twins, one breast can become an ice pack for an overheated baby while the other one mimics a hot-water bottle, should her sister be feeling the chill. We are encouraged to believe a mother's body to be mad and clever and possessed of subtle magic entirely independent of our own conscious knowledge (though it is hard to escape the obvious retort that mine was not quite mad and clever enough to sustain a pregnancy). Fathers also calm an infant and promote weight gain, but cannot perform this thermostatic trick, and so in order to cool themselves down babies will often fling an arm up out of the blanket, as if in urgent answer to a question.

Shuffling back and forth from the bathroom in their faded hospital robes, even the fathers here are reduced to patients, dressed up in their sterile glad rags in preparation for a snatched rendezvous. Gabe and I have watched them with envy.

But now Baby A, or A-lette, to use her new diminutive, has been stable for a few hours. Her nurse, Raakhi, asks, would I like to hold her? I am not allowed to lift or carry my daughter, for this must be done by experts, like handling Chihuly glass. But I can, she explains, lie back in a chair and wait for her to be delivered, positioned as if I am an altar.

Day Three

A-lette is anchored at several points. She has a thick hose emerging from her CPAP mask, providing pressurised air and oxygen, and kept on by a truthfully unstylish white cotton hat. On her right foot is a glowing red saturation probe, monitoring the oxygen in her blood. She has an intravenous cannula in her left wrist delivering nutrients and antibiotics, splinted in place with a sort of Styrofoam flip-flop that has been Velcroed over her whole forearm, making it too heavy for her to lift. Her oral-gastric tube emerges from her mouth and is taped to her left cheek. Capped off between feeds, it now hangs loose, about ten inches long. A-lette comes with a tangle of wires and each must be lifted as a piece with her, so as not to pull at her rice-paper skin. Raakhi lowers the side of the incubator and takes some time arranging these cables.

I lie down and we check the lock on the wheels of the chair; then we check it again. I part the folds of my hospital gown: it is like offering up my heart for sacrifice. Tears are sliding silently down my temples and into my ears. And then there is a hot frog on my chest, a handful of human, and Raakhi is expertly folding up her legs, arranging my hand in a firm cup beneath her bent knees. Premature babies crave enclosure, the womb's approximation, now they can no longer have the womb. Space to flail distresses them: in the right way on my chest, Raakhi tells me, I can contain her better than her nest of towels. We check the monitors anxiously, but so far her oxygen and heart rate remain stable. Raakhi is smiling, satisfied. And I am holding one of my daughters.

Across the room while this is happening Sophie is here with her husband, Evan, who is slim and bespectacled, and has the air of a distracted intellectual. They are huddled, whispering together. Until yesterday, Gabe thought Evan was one of the doctors, for he stands poring over William's hospital notes for hours, speaking softly to the nurses and asking question after question, clearly an expert. But it turns out he is only a specialist in William. I did not say hello to Sophie this morning, nor she to me, and I don't know whether this is because it isn't done to talk at the bedsides, or whether we will simply never speak to one another again. It's true that I have never seen her acknowledge Sunny in this room, though in the milking shed they chat. I am learning the rules. I will have to wait to bump into Sophie out there to find out.

In my recliner I am trying to stay calm so that the heart that beats beneath my daughter is the beat that was once familiar to her, slow and steady. But in this position I can't see her, and I ache to study the new person tucked beneath my chin. She is a person I have longed to know. I cannot move, nor can I lower her into my arms, for these babies cannot be held like babies. *I can't see her face*, I whisper to Gabe, over and over. *I can't see her face*. I stare at the wall, at the blinking monitors, at the empty incubator, and try to imagine her. I am overwhelmed with feelings I don't yet understand. Now as I lie here, I am grateful that we parents pretend not to see one another in this room, so our happiness and pain remain our own. What solitude I will have with my daughters can look only like this: meted out and supervised by medical experts, overlooked by Evan and Sophie, Sunny and Sunny's mother. To be blind to one another is essential.

And so I am startled when I see Sophie confer with her husband, who then crosses the nursery to us. Evan is extremely tall: as I lie in my chair, he looms impossibly far above, though he does not even glance down at me, exposed and still weeping. He passes something to Gabe and then he is gone, back to the other side of the room, back to his son, back to pretending that he cannot hear our most intimate murmuring. Gabe closes my fingers around a handle, and I realise that what Sophie has given me is a mirror. If I raise it I can see my daughter's face.

*

It is midnight and Sophie and I are in the milking shed, milking, talking. Our breast pumps click and whirr. The milk drips and splashes, an unavoidably intimate sound. Relations between us have moved at lightning speed: already we have begun to speak of the betrothal of her son William to my daughter A-lette – William's and A-lette's incubators are opposite one another on the ward, so surely it is predestined. At present the combined weight of bride and groom is less than that of a wedding cake, but the joke has nonetheless taken root. Sophie and I were strangers at lunchtime; this evening we are already family. It helps, to imagine our children might have a future together. It helps, to imagine our children might have a future.

When we finish, Sophie leaves to go home and, still myself an inpatient, I go on to the ward. But instead of the silence I had expected, I have come upon a scene.

A-lette's incubator is thrown open and bathed in a pool of white light; six or seven people encircle her so I can see only their backs, and not the baby who lies between them. From the doorway it looks like the ritual of a secret society is being enacted or, what the room has actually become, an operating

42

theatre. The nurse practitioner at the centre wears a headlamp and a look of intense concentration. One of the others spots me and breaks away.

You can't be in here now. She glances back impatiently towards the others; she does not have time for me, nor for the note of terror audible in my voice when I ask what is happening. *We're running a central line, to help your baby take in calories. It takes a long time, you won't want to wait; we've had to start all over again.*

It's clear from her expression that she immediately regrets this last statement as, far from disappearing as she intended, I am standing rigid, waiting for her to explain. *We got the first one all the way into position and it was faulty, the guide wire wouldn't come out. We had to start all over again. Your other daughter's one went in okay*, she adds. A note of criticism is detectable in her voice, though criticism of what or whom I cannot fathom.

I am dismissed, left, frozen, in the hallway. If my child is having a procedure, shouldn't I be there? Or here, waiting just outside for its conclusion? Shouldn't I at least have known it was happening? Or maybe they did tell me and I didn't understand – that is entirely possible. A junior doctor is writing notes at the nurses' station, and looks up.

Didn't you know they were doing it tonight?

I shake my head tightly, and so he sets down his pen and explains that these babies will not be able to feed themselves for a long time, and I wonder as he says this whether this is the first time I have heard it overtly stated. Intravenous cannulas – IVs – are good for quick dextrose and medication but they are not very stable, and need replacing every few days. The doctors need a longer-term channel to deliver nutrition. And so a central line, a longline, will run from her ankle through her veins, and all the way to her heart.

Why are there so many people in there?

He begins to straighten the lanyard of his hospital ID. He is so young that he still resembles the young man in the photograph, pink-cheeked and curly-haired. He frowns down at himself. There is no pain relief given for the procedure, he explains. The nurses who stand in attendance are pinning down the baby.

Upstairs, Gabe and I sit side by side in silence, each of us on Google Scholar, but we can find no good reason why neonates are not given analgesics for procedures known to hurt. Several articles conclude that it is hard to calculate the correct dose for a very tiny baby and that errors would be dangerous; but just because something is hard does not mean it ought not to be done.

We learn that there was, for many years, a belief that premature babies were unable to feel pain due to the immaturity of their nervous systems, just as, for many years, the same was believed of animals. This reassuring fallacy about infant pain perception has been hard to upend, in the same way people once resisted the roundness of the world. The knowledge changes everything.

It's possible that neonatologists do not want to think about the suffering they inflict with their decisions, and with their hands. Work, for them, would be easier, believing that they practise their arts not on babies but on pre-babies; phantoms who will graduate into full babydom only once their medical requirements have ended. No agony or loneliness. It is hard and very painful to believe that premature babies are people, and for that sort of pain there is no analgesic except denial. I understand why they might deny it. They suffer, too, the doctors.

In fact, the latest research suggests that babies feel pain more, not less, acutely than adults. On the glowing screen of Gabe's phone, from April of this year, *fMRI reveals neural activity overlap between adult and infant pain*; or from the journal *Neonatology* in February of last year, my own phone wonders more bluntly, *Eight Years Later, Are We Still Hurting Newborn Infants?*

Is this research too new to have reached clinical practice? Or must the team downstairs, at present pinning down my daughter, have their own reasons? They must, they must! From the fold-out chair on which he has taken to sleeping, beside my own hospital bed, Gabe grips my hand a little too tightly.

It felt as if the nurse who barred my entrance was angry with me, for my inconvenient questions, for my inconvenient feelings. I wonder if these tired medics in their headlamps, those who have spent an hour carefully positioning a central line they then have to remove, ever find themselves angry with the babies for the failure of the guide wire, for the failure of equipment that took place within those babies' veins. I wonder if they cover up the face of the child into whose body they must work thirty centimetres of silicone, painstaking millimetre by millimetre, and whether, when it is a second attempt and very late, some might be tempted to go just a little faster than they ought.

DAY FOUR

Tuesday, 6th October

The women I pass, faceless before, are shimmering into individuality. Daniella, who is a teaching assistant in a girls' school. She had her daughter Atlanta when she was very young; now her sixteen-year-old is a perfect doppelgänger, with the same arched eyebrows and long dark hair, the same ready smile. Responsible and serious, Atlanta comes every day after school to visit her new little brother, Phoenix, who was born unexpectedly at twenty-eight weeks. Even at sixteen, it cannot be easy to relinquish your mother to these long NICU days. Phoenix can still only come out of his incubator once a day, but several times a week Daniella gives her cuddle – Cuddle – to Atlanta.

Jess, whose son, Rafi, was born two days after the girls, only twenty-six weeks but with a full head of astonishing red hair. Yesterday Jess and I compared our various minor discomforts while we expressed, and she has since won my life-long gratitude by dispatching her husband Pete to buy us each some nipple cream. I had not yet met Pete but he slipped a tube to me wordlessly in the locker room this morning, without eye contact, like a dealer.

Kemisha is a pack leader here, among us mothers of the Neonatal Intensive Care Unit. Another veteran, Kemisha is a startling beauty, with an unexpected and effortless glamour entirely at odds with this intrinsically unglamorous place. Kemisha carries the invisible decoration of the soldier who has been to the brink, the Victoria Cross of NICU motherhood. Her daughter, Evanee, was just twenty-four weeks when she was born, close to the legal line of viability. If Sophie looks young to me Kemisha is younger still: maybe in the first years of her twenties. How are these children coping with their sick children, I keep thinking? At thirty-five and thirty-seven, and after eight years together, Gabe and I are – supposedly – adults. Kemisha and her husband Tom were newlyweds when they conceived, and just five and a half months later they were sitting beside an incubator, their 680g daughter not expected to live.

What was I doing in my early twenties? I was single; I was working as a features writer at *Tatler*; I was in £10 sky-high heels from New Look, carrying an enormous inflatable shark around the Serpentine summer party, given the spectacularly silly charge of photographing it with Damien Hirst, or Damien Hirst with it. I was not shouting at doctors; I was certainly not watching a soul I'd made, in peril.

I don't know from what deep source she draws her confidence, but Kemisha feels entitled to attention here. Entitled to be taken seriously, to be heard. She is vivid with a furious, and furiously-channelled, confidence. She embodies the persona we should all be assuming now, here: mother lion, obsessive medical autodidact. Evanee means 'young fighter' but that just as well describes Kemisha. The rest of us shape our days around the morning ward rounds, when we listen and glean and read between lines, thankful to be included, and to ask our tentative questions only when the consultant has finished briefing the nurses and junior doctors for whom the ward round is actually intended. Kemisha – how has she done it? – has had meetings with consultants elsewhere, in offices, behind desks. She doesn't feel the need to appease or apologise, her only focus is that Evanee gets the best care. My approach is establishing itself as quite the opposite: I cannot shake my need to be liked, and to be seen as appropriately grateful to the hard-working staff who have been literally keeping our children alive, hour to hour. My plan, if I can be said to have one, is to kill them with kindness, with reasonableness, to be all honey with no trace of vinegar. Beside Kemisha, who is more than ten years younger than I am, I feel myself infantile, and ignorant.

Sophie and I are pumping again, but we are no longer wedding planning because I am asking Sophie advice. The last hours have not been good ones and that, this week, is really saying something. A-lette has had a suspected infection, and has been nil by mouth yet again, pumped full of a nuclear-strength trio of intravenous antibiotics, until an X-ray revealed that her feeding tube had slipped down too low, into her duodenum. She was bloated, mottled and struggling to breathe because the nurses had been flooding her bowel with milk once an hour. We too have been flooding her bowel with milk, in fact, for this morning Gabe and I were taught how to feed our children – by holding aloft a tiny syringe of milk in the manner of Lady Liberty with her torch, for it to drip down their oral-gastric tubes, straight into their stomachs.

Sophie and I have been discussing this for some time when Kemisha lets herself into the milking shed behind us and begins setting up, wiping disinfectant on the pump, expertly connecting tubes and bottles, unhooking her bra. She and I have not yet spoken, though I have somehow absorbed her story. I continue to Sophie – should I say anything to the doctors? Kemisha doesn't look up. *Someone's fucked up*, she says succinctly. *Those NG tubes have clear measurements printed on them. You should make a fuss.*

From Kemisha and so many other women I will learn, but these lessons will be painful, and slow. I do not make a fuss on this or several other occasions. For now I am simply exhausted with gratitude and relief that it was a slipped feeding tube and not Necrotising Enterocolitis, NEC, which kills premature babies on NICU wards with sinister regularity. NEC had been the likely candidate until the clarifying, incriminating X-ray.

Many months later I will ask my dear friend Adam, an obstetrician at another hospital, whose children he thought would have received better care, mine or Kemisha's. She all fire and fight; I, all obsequious gratitude. In my kitchen, over a Chinese takeaway, Adam will admonish, *The NHS cares for all its patients equally, Francesca*. And then after a pause, *But ... almost certainly hers.*

*

A-lette is awake, eyes open. Her face is turned towards my voice, though I know she cannot see me. She is unable to focus, and her pupils can't yet constrict to protect her retinas in bright light. In any case, the huge mask and CPAP hose upon her face wouldn't do much for the view.

She is on her back in a deep nest of bright banana yellow. She has a longline in one foot now so I cannot touch it, but I hold the other one steady to provide a reassuring boundary against which she can push, evoking the containing muscle of a womb. My palm looks true, shocking white beneath her long red toes, but their pressure upon the base of my thumb is surprisingly strong. No fat but muscle, then. Her white hospital identity bands lie curled in the corner of the incubator. Her skin does not have the integrity to tolerate them, so we must trust the nurses not to pull any Gilbert and Sullivan switches.

I've been discharged, I tell her. *There's nowhere for me to stay here any more.* I don't know how I expect her to respond to this development. I suppose that I want her to be quite clear that mine is not a voluntary abandonment. Am I asking for her understanding? Her forgiveness?

I want to whisper, *One day soon you will both come home with us*, but I don't know if that is the truth. Certainly I have no right or authority to promise.

When she is finally asleep I lift my hands from her with t'ai chi slowness. I approach B-lette's incubator, but the nurse shakes her head. The baby is settled now, and she does not think I should disturb her, simply to take my leave. For the first time since my daughters' birth I step with Gabe from the elevator out into the lobby, and onwards, towards the late-night commerce of the nearby high street. With each move away from them I feel myself grow heavier until, by the time Gabe pulls up at our front door, it is all that I can do to put one foot in front of the other. Home is now the NICU, the only place in which my family can be together. I feel as if I have left my daughters exposed upon a hillside.

Four days ago I left behind a crime scene, but Gabe has mopped the bathroom floor and, I presume, thrown away the sheets. We move through the remaining stages of the evening as fast as possible; we bolt down a shepherd's pie from my sister that appeared, as if by magic, while we were at the hospital; then I tackle the stairs with steady determination while Gabe does the washing-up. I arrive in our bedroom to find a bunch of burnt-orange tulips beside a newly rented breast pump, which has itself been adorned: a Fudge bar is in one of its small bottle-holders, and a miniature packet of Jelly Babies is in the other. For the sake of efficiency I do as much of my crying as possible in the shower, then I crawl under the covers while downstairs Gabe snatches a few moments to answer his most pressing work emails. I have no idea when he found time to do all this. I don't know how it is he knows instinctively when to help and when to leave me to a fight of my own, but he senses whenever I need the reassurance of my own self-sufficiency. I am grateful he did not offer to help me up the stairs, though I am certain he would have preferred simply to carry me. In return, I will not ask him how he's feeling, as I know that he will not want to have to consider the answer.

Eventually Gabe comes upstairs to bed where I am sprawled, waiting for him like a bad joke, in a parody of lingerie: giant parachute knickers, deafening conical breast pump. When I have finished this round he runs the milk downstairs to the fridge while in the bathroom sink I scrub plastic parts to be ready again in the small hours.

What I need now more than anything is to be able to curl on my side, pressed close against my husband. The warmth of his skin on mine is the greatest sedative, the surest way I've ever known to calm my mind, to steady my pulse. For the last months of my pregnancy I have slept upright in order to breathe, peering down at Gabe with sorrowful myopia as at a world far below, like looking into a valley over the handrail of a bridge. To once again sleep next to him was the only consolation of this move home, but I find I cannot lie on my side for the strain on my incision, and cannot fill my lungs with his arm across my chest. So I lie flat on my back and clutch his hand like a lifeline. I am fascinated and appalled by the remaining slack pouch of flesh where a hundred hours ago I housed our daughters. In the dark I touch it, gingerly. This is where they still should be, beneath the covers, beneath my skin, palpable and distant, drawing slowly closer to us like a ship from the horizon. Where, now, do they believe themselves to be?

I have visited the mothers of newborns. I have seen their fatigue, their distraction, their longing for just a breath of liberty from this new consuming tyranny. But I remember too that when a helpful friend takes the child from their arms, that stunned and softened look will sharpen, replaced by one of hunger, and an urge to snatch back the baby they have only moments ago offered with relief. I have seen their jealousy, a fleeting separation seductive and intolerable.

When I am apart from my daughters, my physical pain becomes almost incapacitating. I wonder which is real – its fading to a meaningless background hum in their presence or now, like this, its raging grip in their absence. All day I am on my feet, walking, opening and closing the drawers beneath the incubator, sitting, standing, bending. At night all motion stops and into the void rushes sensation: burning, vivid, essential, but oddly referred. I feel it not in my abdomen but as an endless spasm in my lower back, and a whiplash tension in my shoulders and neck. Perhaps it is a blessing, distracting me from everything else that hurts.

DAY FIVE

Wednesday, 7th October

I am a new mother learning to change a wet nappy, an everyday rite of passage. I peer down through the top of the incubator, with one arm through each porthole. The task ahead feels like performing a cross between keyhole surgery and a puppet show. But this will be my fourth; surely I will have made some improvement.

All manipulations of premature babies involve a multitude of factors. They must be handled like precious relics, like the irreplaceably old. Each move must be calculated and cautious, gentle as an art restorer working on a Vermeer.

From each foot runs a tube or wire; on the baby's left foot the glowing saturation probe, the light shining hot through her translucent foot like the red glow of a slow-sinking evening sun. Into her right ankle runs the hated, necessary longline: somewhere in that fatless leg it ascends, almost to the chambers of her heart. From her left hand emerges an intravenous cannula for medication and glucose. On her bare chest are three sticky squares from which finer leads emerge, monitoring her temperature, heart and respiration rate. The nurses gather these three into a neat bouquet and tape them down with one tab of the nappy, to keep them from tangling.

With Raakhi's encouragement I use the flat of my hand beneath the baby's knees and thighs to push them back as gently as I can, and it is as if, in lifting her knees, I have opened a faucet. Perhaps I have compressed something in the baby's tummy because suddenly there is an expulsion of poo, mustard yellow, coming with such unexpected trajectory and force it is as if someone stepped on an open tube of toothpaste. It is on the front and back of both of my hands, and smeared down both wrists. It is on the sheets, and on the monitoring electrodes. It is still squirting from the baby but I don't even know how to begin to stop it. I have moved a hundred miles beyond my competency, and beyond any hope of resolution. I can only wait, like a castaway bobbing on a raft. If Raakhi doesn't put her hands through the other side to help I will be trapped like this for ever. I begin turning from left to right and back again as I search hopelessly for a solution, when I see Raakhi beside me, her hand clapped over her mouth. *It's on her hat*, is all she manages, and then succumbs to helpless giggles.

*

The women of the milking shed have begun to bring me names, after I told them what the nurse threatened yesterday – that the staff will choose for the babies soon, if we don't. *We had some twins who were Tom and Jerry within the week. Can't even remember what the parents called them in the end but it didn't matter, they were too slow, so we took matters into our own hands. Tom and Jerry. Cute little ones, they were.*

Yesterday, Lisa looked with pity at my *Penguin Book of Baby Names*, 1995 Edition. It was clear from her expression she did not think I was going to find anything sensible from a year in which we'd all worn muddy brown lipstick and feathered bobs, so today she came in with her own paperbacks, complete with highlighted greatest hits. She knew long ago her daughter would be Emma, though she also considered Nicole, which is now up for grabs. Kemisha had no backup names – her daughter was Evanee, instantly and completely. Daniella knew early that Phoenix was a boy. Everyone likes Vivienne, and we all love Violet, which Kemisha gave to Evanee as a middle name. The room is hotly divided on whether identical twins should or should not begin with the same letter. A mother I don't recognise, down here in red flannel pyjamas printed with candy canes and gingerbread men, weighs in. *Well, I just had an emergency hysterectomy on Friday getting Jason out, didn't I, so I ain't having another girl now.* She gives a short dry bark of laughter, before offering me Grace, a name she'd saved, and treasured.

*

A-lette has a wound on her right hand that isn't healing. We are asked to sign consent forms for Medical Photography to come and take records. No one explains, but it becomes clear that this damage, a site of florid bruising from which her fine skin has flayed, is from a cannula inserted badly, or possibly a cannula inserted correctly that the baby herself has decided to displace. They have only been alive since Friday but Babies A and B have accumulated a collection of raw puncture wounds, and as a layman I cannot see the difference between the one that concerns the nurses and the other ones that do not. Still, I sign the form.

The photographer comes, a pale, nervous man in his early forties, formally dressed, who seems anxious to get this over with. In these last days I have become acutely sensitive to what I can only wincingly call people's 'energies' – he has said very little, but I wish he would calm down. Round his neck is a long-lensed digital SLR, such as a paparazzo might carry. He needs us to open up the incubator. Also he would like to use a very bright flash, and how do we think the baby might feel about it? The baby, I tell him, would not feel at all good about such a flash. He nods, but cannot see a way around it. Shall we cover her face? Yes, that seems a good idea. I pull her knitted hat down over her eyes but the purl separates, so this will be insufficient. The nurse suggests a nappy. My daughters wear nappies in a size substantially smaller than the commercial size 0, they wear the smallest size, in fact, in production. Still, we must fold them down to fit. One of these diminutive sanitary items is procured and arranged on A-lette's head. *I'm sorry*, I whisper, genuinely apologetic. This humiliation seems a final insult. The photographer adjusts his settings. At the last moment the nurse pushes a button, and the top of the incubator disengages, whirring upwards like a space ship. Baby A and her damaged right arm are exposed to gusts of cold air and bright white flashes, and then it is all over and the lid whirrs down again. Through the porthole I remove the nappy from her head. I apologise to her further though she refuses to respond to my overture, and I can hardly blame her.

Across the room Sophie is watching in silence, forming her own conclusions. Already I feel I have always known her, but only this morning did she and I get around to revealing what we each do for a living. It felt almost fanciful to speak of anything outside the walls of this hospital, to discuss the outside world, in which Sophie is a senior executive at a charity that campaigns internationally for women's rights, and in which my own half-finished novel has receded to unimaginable remoteness, as if viewed down the wrong end of a telescope. Later Sophie will induce my first stitch-straining belly laugh of NICU when she tells me she presumed that A-lette's photo shoot was a result of my fame as an author. It's possible that Sophie needs to adjust her expectations about the publishing of literary novels.

*

The milking shed is in quorum when I arrive. Eloise and Sophie are in the cockpit, craning around backwards. Behind them in the cabin are Daniella and Kemisha – my arrival makes it crowded in our little craft. The pumps are all taken but Kemisha already has one full bottle of milk in her lap, so it can't be long before she finishes. I sit down in the circle to wait. Eloise is talking loudly.

The thing is, it's just making me fucking miserable, she is saying, craning around to address the others. Everyone is nodding, faces grave. *It's been nine weeks. I just worked it out; it's sixty-five days now.*

I study a faint bleach stain on the knee of my tracksuit bottoms, grateful that I did not burst in with my ignorance, with my questions, with my *newness*. Eloise's son Henry was born at what should have been a respectable thirty-five weeks but has had a tumbling dominoes series of complications, setback after setback.

I just thought it would be so much quicker than this. Eloise's voice catches, and I feel my own throat constrict with hers. Everyone is nodding, heartfelt, sympathetic. They are heroines here. They are warriors. Eloise pats her stomach. *Nine weeks and I still can't fucking zip them up.*

Sophie shakes her head. She is eating a chocolate Penguin. *Nine months on, nine months off,* she says, and around the room everyone is nodding their assent. With her mouth full she adds, *Or in Kemisha's case, five months on, five months off. Good thinking, K.*

Kemisha grins. *Exactly, it's your own fault.* She detaches her second bottle and screws on the lilac lid. Her nails are painted in a slightly darker, shimmering shade. *I don't know what you were all thinking, being pregnant so bloody long.*

Immediately outside this door are the lockers where other parents are clocking in or clocking out, removing watches and wedding rings. I wonder what they will make of the full-throated, indecent, intemperate laughter. Our greatest gift to one another is this: each woman of the milking shed has been swept out by a riptide, pulled far from the current of normal motherhood. Apart and all together in this space, our odd craft, we are drawn back into the folds of the unremarkable.

DAY SIX

Thursday, 8th October

Leaving my children each night is an amputation, over and over.

Yet there is a pervasive sense that we are not yet entitled to stake our full claim upon them. In the NICU we are considered less necessary than we would be on the paediatric wards, for when real children are admitted to hospital there is usually an adult cot beside their hospital bed, in which a mother or father will stay. Is that what it is, that these aren't yet real children? Or is it that we aren't yet real parents?

When I wake at 2 a.m. I pump for precisely twenty-six minutes. I phone the ward for a whispered update – A-lette had a green aspirate that was not returned to her stomach; B-lette's aspirate was milky, which is good. They will be weighed shortly, which no one enjoys. Instead of passing the bottle to a nurse as I could when I was an inpatient I must now rouse Gabe for him to put the milk in the fridge, downstairs. Each time he hushes me when I say sorry and try to reassure him that soon, surely, I will be well enough to do it myself. *It is a chance to say hello to you*, he says. There is so little he can do for our daughters. At least with my endless expressing I can convince myself, at a stretch, that even my own breakfast is in their service. He hurts my heart, bounding downstairs without his glasses, climbing back into bed so carefully so as not to shift the mattress and cause me a jolt of discomfort. After a while I will hear his breath change and hope that in sleep he is relieved of worry, for a while.

I know that we are lucky to live so close to the hospital. But still. Though my pain is now a steady, thrumming four, the trips there and back are a particular trial. It is as if every speed bump has been aligned en route, every corner sharpened. With each slalom I lower my head and wrap my arms around the loose mound of my belly, to clamp it in place. The sensation is one of momentum, of swinging a bag of fine membrane from which my organs might burst at the crest of a sharp turn. Whatever inner scaffolding I once had has been dismantled and I am held together but barely. I cannot yet even think about the bus. *Please,* I say weakly, to Uber driver after Uber driver as we hurtle down the main road, *please, I have just had surgery*.

To rest I now have only the milking shed, and access to the parents' kitchen, which contains a mini fridge plastered with signs exhorting us to 'PLEASE LABEL AND DATE YOUR FOOD' and, sometimes, an open packet of pink wafer biscuits beside the kettle. I have never taken one, as I can't determine whether or not they are communal. Several times I have been in this kitchen to find a father taking a lengthy work call – the men seem to feel this is the place for business, often standing with their foreheads to the window, shutting out the distinctly unprofessional reality behind them, frowning down into the traffic, or pacing the room on a headset, gesticulating with a polystyrene coffee cup. I do not go there often.

During the day, the endless pumping is an essential tyranny. I keep being told it is the most important thing I can do for my daughters; but as the nurses urge me back towards the milking shed, I feel as if I am being shooed from under their feet, and being told to go and play in the traffic. My only relief is to be touching my babies, if only with a fingertip.

The mornings are the hardest, when I have been longest from my children.

The nights are the hardest, when the longest stretch without them lies ahead.

*

My milk is in. In the shower it comes, unmistakable, overwhelming. As women we are unused to autonomous body parts; mostly our bodies move only as we will them, or they alter with imperceptible, lunar slowness. But this sudden swell is urgent; it comes like the surge and heat of a geyser; like monsoon rain. My body has finally understood. Tears of relief mingle with the falling water.

DAY SEVEN

Friday, 9th October

I have become a leaflet reader; a helpline caller. I have become the recipient of charity, in several forms:

1. Hats. Both my children wear hats, on heads not much larger than snooker balls. They are regularly described in the hospital notes (*Ms B-lette Segal was seen cavorting in style, sporting a stylish beanie in blue and pink stripes*), because for hygiene purposes they must be changed regularly, like their oxygen masks, like their NG tubes, like their bedding. These hats are not only functional but beautiful, and they are hand-knitted by generous women whose inspiration and

motivation I cannot imagine. These women knit hats in many sizes, and many sizes smaller than those worn by my daughters. They knit beautiful, cabled hats for babies whose birth is recorded simply as 'late miscarriage'. They knit soft hats for babies who never took a breath. I imagine them assembled in a church hall, the flash and clack of needles, refilling their cups from the hissing tea urn, these good women gossiping about their grandchildren and their azaleas and their plans for the Christmas Fayre, these women who are not afraid to think of or knit for death.

2. Dummies. They can't suck them yet, but beside each of my girls, a dolly-sized pacifier has appeared. They can practise sucking, and will derive comfort from the exercise of this reflex. Dummies are also believed to prevent babies from slipping into too deep a sleep, and thereby forgetting to breathe.

3. Our own mirrors. Indigo folding pocket mirrors, one for each child, to prevent cross-contamination. We caused uproar, apparently, borrowing William's larger one, though if he and A-lette are to be married I see no reason for such modesty.

4. Memory boxes. At some point over the last hours, memory boxes have arrived. These are very large, baby pink shoeboxes, each containing a notepad and pen, a small book of nursery rhymes, a knot of coloured felt rope that my

daughters will apparently one day enjoy grasping, and a baby-pink ink pad together with a piece of thick creamy card for taking hand and footprints. It is hard to state how much I loathe this last item, the ink pad. There is such kindness here, and generosity of spirit. Kindness, time, money. But while they cling so determinedly to life I will not memorialise them. I do not want my children contained within a memory box, with all that that implies. The box itself is an evocative, ominous size.

5. Zaky hands. These are creepy or wonderful or heartbreaking, or some indecipherable muddle of the three. Zaky hands are life-size disembodied beanbag hands in a variety of Easter-egg pastel shades, designed solely and specifically to bring comfort and reassurance to premature babies. Each of my children has been given a fuzzy lilac one. I was encouraged to nestle these for several hours in my bra so that they would take on my scent. At home last night we ate my father-in-law's renowned roast chicken, while down my maternity vest reached two plush purple arms, as if I was being felt up by a Muppet. Nothing seems strange to us any more, perhaps because everything is strange. Their weight and retained heat is similar to a human hand and so whenever I am expressing or sleeping the Zakys will lie across our babies'

backs, and our babies will feel held, and safe. I feel unbounded gratitude to the anonymous donor of these hands, which retail at $99 a pair and must be shipped in from Australia, though of course if we didn't have to leave our daughters night after night, no hands but our own would be required.

All of this is quite apart from the unquestioned and unquestioning egalitarian compassion of the National Health Service. I have read of American families losing jobs, selling homes, forced to weigh and value every scan, every test and medication against the financial ruin to follow.

Gabe and I have both been exceptionally lucky: until last week, neither of us had spent a night in hospital since our own births. But the National Health Service has been here for us all along nonetheless, invisible in its familiarity, too old, too lumbering to win the songs of gratitude and romance it deserves. In good times it goes all but unnoticed, like the hard invisible work of a loving parent, mentioned only in articles decrying understaffed departments, long waiting lists. And of course the NHS is, like all human constructions, imperfect. But its sheer moral courage as an endeavour makes it an institution of which we should be inordinately proud. It is a monument to means-blind, universal compassion, and to goodness.

Their ministrations to each of my daughters cost in the region of two thousand pounds per twenty-four-hour period. It has already been a week, world-class care for which I will never be presented with, nor ever even see, a bill.

*

Sophie is on the warpath. *There is someone in the parents' kitchen brazenly mixing a Lemsip. Lemsip! If you need Lemsip, GO HOME!*

We text furiously back and forth, increasingly outraged, ostensibly with the selfishness of the Lemsip-sipping mother but really the fury is with ourselves. Sophie stayed silent while the woman shook out her sachet and brewed her treacherous telltale paracetamol, and I know I would have done the same. Kemisha, we agree, would have said something. It might have made no difference; surely she already knew she shouldn't have come to the ward. But perhaps it was simply that no one had explained the rules: *You are not allowed to be sick here. You are not allowed to be sick or needy or distracted or bored or dispirited or angry or noisy or high-strung, you are allowed to be neither demanding nor too passive. While you are here you must be perfect.* Come on, lady. It's really not a lot to ask.

73

DAY EIGHT

Saturday, 10th October

A-lette is mottled and bloated; her abdomen looks taut and shiny as a balloon, and her brow is furrowed with obvious discomfort. The nurse became anxious when her oxygen requirement went up for the third time and paged the registrar, who also doesn't like what he sees. A-lette is floppy and lethargic. He prescribes intravenous ceftazidime and teicoplanin. She is once again nil by mouth. He thinks she has a longline infection.

We have begun to understand the risks of prematurity, but the staff rarely speak of the risks of intervention. It is

Sophie who tells me, *Did you know that Stevie Wonder, born six weeks early, was blinded by the oxygen given to save his life?* No one speaks to us of much; we are not consulted. Perhaps there was no time, or perhaps, most likely, there was no choice. The longline was a necessary invasion, for their unready guts can barely digest and certainly cannot take in enough nourishment to survive. Why dwell upon the risks of the essential? And so I hadn't known, but quite apart from the horror of insertion, a longline is a constant, mid-level anxiety for a baby's caregivers, offering an open channel for infection, right into the very centre of the child. Bacteria that enter here will find a smooth passage, all the way into her heart.

Perhaps it is good that we are told so little; perhaps there is a plan at work here, in the management of our understanding, and we are given gobbets of information as it is believed we could cope with them. Day by day I feel a painstaking accretion of my understanding and yet still my experience is of a series of unpleasant surprises sprung, one after another, just when we have begun to assimilate the consequences of the last. It does not seem possible to see a complete laundry list of all the things that can go wrong here, though I feel it would calm me in some perverse way, were someone to present me with such a document. I would like to see the size of all we face, to feel its telephone directory weight. We know to fear NEC and brain bleeds. We know that lung damage is likely or at least possible; we know they may not see or hear like other children.

We know their bowels are struggling, and their immune systems are ill-equipped for the daily invisible interchange of filth, given and received, consumed and inhaled, that is life in a human city. With my own antibodies in my breast milk I can at least fortify them against the bacteria to which I myself am exposed, a thought that makes me want to drink from every abandoned coffee cup in Starbucks; to kiss sneezing strangers; to lick the high street pavements.

Now the longline, run to save my child, might be poisoning her. A state of openness is always a state of vulnerability. Yet I watch her laboured breath and I cannot help it: I feel love coursing and burning through every vein and artery, though I understand that through the open channel I am inviting devastation.

DAY NINE

Sunday, 11th October

Each day I come to peer at my children in an extremely well-funded prison or perhaps more accurately a high-tech zoo, at which privileged visitors are permitted to interact with the exhibits. After the horror of yesterday A-lette seems much better today, responding to the antibiotics, and so the longline remains, though now I eye it in her incubator like a snake, coiled and waiting to strike. I want it out, but obviously that isn't possible while she is nil by mouth, for it is her only source of nutrition. Brave little B-lette is marching ever onwards, tiny warrior. She gained six grams last night.

That is a teaspoonful, but around here we celebrate every sachet of sugar.

B-lette was awake when I arrived and so I held her, lying back in my wipe-clean, grape-coloured plastic recliner, her body on mine, featherweight. We breathe together, and I breathe my wishes into her, my lips against the purple crochet of her hat. Yesterday was not good, she and I agree. Today will be better.

When I move to the milking shed Sophie is in the cockpit, with someone I don't recognise beside her as co-pilot. They are already talking and so I lift a hand in a silent greeting, and get on with setting up my pump behind them. I am in need of Sophie's counsel. The consultant on this morning's ward round said that it was likely we would soon be transferred to our 'Local', as if the next hospital were a pub to which we might mosey for a quiet pint on a Sunday evening.

It becomes clear that, as a world centre, this is a field hospital – when you are fit to travel they will patch you up and send you on, in order to make way for those who cannot be cared for elsewhere – the tinies, the hopeless cases, the future miracles. Our designated 'Local' is a few miles closer to home, though until today I had barely heard of it and had no idea where it was. Apparently it is a crumbling former smallpox hospital. To get there our children will be starved and hyper-caffeinated, loaded into a portable incubator and then an ambulance. I would like Sophie to coax me down from a very high branch of anxiety, like a fireman with a cat, but I have to set all that aside, for now. William had a crucial eye examination this morning, and I want to ask her how it went.

The woman talking to Sophie has a baby in Nursery Five. Her son has been here a week now and she hopes that he is going home tomorrow, or the next day. She has a very flippy blonde ponytail, worn high, like a cheerleader. She seems full of the joys of spring. Sophie must know her a little for she refers to the woman's son by name, and asks how the breastfeeding is going. *Great, thank goodness, the lactation woman says he's got a great latch, which is why I'm not getting in here as much, but I figured I'd keep up the pumping a bit, you know, just so we have some in the freezer and my partner can do the odd night. That's why I'm glad that he went in to work this week, so he can take his parental leave next week, when we're home.* She crunches on a carrot stick, and I realise that the scent of garlic in the small room is emanating from a small pot of hummus open on the table in front of her. *Why is Evan using his parental leave now, didn't you want to save it?*

In profile, I watch Sophie's expression. *You don't owe her an answer*, I think, feeling my own face flush. *Just say any old thing*, but Sophie offers the truth. *Because now is when we have William. He might never come home.* I study the other woman for signs of embarrassment and find none. I am perfectly positioned behind them – I could so easily bash her on the head with the *Penguin Book of Names*, 1995 Edition, like Whack-a-Mole, and she would never see it coming.

DAY TEN

Monday, 12th October

I have just spotted that there is a sign on the outside door
saying that peanuts are not permitted on the ward, and I am
stricken. For the last three days in a row I have been bringing
in oatcakes smeared with peanut butter (to mask the taste of
the tar-like blackstrap molasses my mother advises is going
to restore my iron levels), and eating these nutritionally-
engineered sandwiches in the milking shed. I was enraged
by the selfish ignorance of the Lemsip woman but I have
been moving around unwittingly like Typhoid Mary,
spreading peanut dust and possible anaphylaxis. I send a

distraught text to Sophie, who replies moments later with a link to a study showing that premature infants have fewer allergies than term babies (how did she find such a thing? An actual advantage of prematurity? Has she forged it?), and another new study from the *New England Journal of Medicine* showing that early exposure to allergens reduces risk of later hypersensitivity. *You basically did everyone here a favour*, she concludes, and I wonder how I would make it through a week here without her. I don't think I'd make it through an hour.

DAY ELEVEN

Tuesday, 13th October

Gabe woke up with a blocked nose and a slight scratch at the back of his throat. In ordinary life it might warrant at most a whiskey and an early night. But in our new reality it is enough to illuminate the lurid hex of a virus upon him, and to bar him admission to the hospital. Either hospital, I should say, for today B-lette will be moving to the Local, four miles up the road. You take beds at your local hospital as they come up; one has come up. One, I should add, not two. The other twin will remain behind until a second space is free, which could be today, or next week, or next month.

I can't, I venture rather tentatively, be in two places at once? This is apparently no one's problem but my own. Meanwhile, the ambulance in which B-lette must travel will siren-scream through roads we should have driven with our newborn babies in a proud and careful silence, a home-coming, months from now. My daughter will almost pass our front door, but she will not be stopping there.

You'll love the Local, nurses keep assuring me, and then invariably add, *but first you'll really hate it*.

Why? Here it is spanking new – new building, new incubators, glossy with new paint and shiny gizmos, generously funded, the corridors washed through with eddying rivers of cash. Those disposable pumping kits – the sterile tubing, the bottles, which we each use, a new one every time, eight to ten times a day – those, I learn, cost ten quid each. At the Local we'll get one kit on arrival and will have to scrub it with a squirt of washing-up liquid and a paper hand towel eight to ten times a day, instead. What sterilising takes place must happen at night, at home, in the steam steriliser I do not yet own. Forget miniature premature dummies for learning to suck, gel pillows to stave off square heads, Zaky hands for positioning and comfort, all of those cost money. At the

Local, they make it sound, the girls will be lucky to have a cardboard box, a pair of fingerless gloves and a space near the brazier. *But the staff are amazing*, I am told over and over, and when in a panic I text my friend Adam, the obstetrician, he is singing from the same hymn sheet. *The building is shite, but parents end up loving the NICU. And the nurses and doctors are the nicest. Say hello to Deepak!* I do not feel inclined to say hello to anyone. I do not want my children in a crumbling former smallpox hospital with no money, and no locker room in which to leave my bag. ITEMS ARE LEFT AT OWNER'S RISK should not be a concern in the place I must leave a child. I am frightened to wash breast pump parts in a ward sink from which I am convinced we will all contract MRSA. And on whose design advice did the hospital administrators decide to position the Neonatal Intensive Care Unit immediately opposite the Tuberculosis Clinic?

Today, still shrinking, B-lette weighed in at a precise, supermarket-worthy 1,000 grams. But she has been deemed the more stable twin and is off on her travels while A-lette remains in situ, close to all the modern conveniences of the town centre. Milk will be needed round the clock in both places. My breasts will have to find a way to split their time.

*

On what I hadn't known would be my final scan before giving birth, the babies were both frank breech. The sonographer pressed her wand into my tight belly and showed us two mirror faces in conference, bolt upright.

Contemporary developmental psychology stresses the need for parents to differentiate monozygotic twins, to acknowledge and encourage their differences. We had already decided not to dress them alike, that one would learn piano and the other karate, that we would avoid confusion with radically different haircuts. Now, gazing at their silent communion I understood the idiocy of making prescriptive plans. A child will not embrace the bassoon because her parents will it; second and more vitally, here are two beings who were once – however briefly – a single being. *This is what you are*, I thought, and vowed to remember. For an hour or a day or anything up to a week I moved through the world pregnant with a single child, a predecessor, or an ancestor, even, a single child who was lost at the moment of their division into their two selves. Before them I carried their genetic clone and she was both and yet, primordial, she was neither. An embryo's splitting into identical twins is for the moment unexplained, and so we will have to say only that they became two for private reasons of their own.

I felt relief when the sonographer's pressure eased and the screen returned to blankness. It was too intimate a union for our clumsy witness, and felt like spying. *In utero* my daughters stood erect like soldiers; nose to nose like puppies; palm to palm through their fine membrane, like the pilgrim Romeo and Juliet.

A nurse, Luciana, suggests, *before they are separated why don't you hold them both together*, and though the sterilising and preparation for such a manoeuvre is as lengthy and complex as for open heart surgery, the surgical gown and the wires and the checks, two nurses, levitating cables to disentangle, oxygen to monitor, limbs and blankets to arrange, once I am in place, heart surgery is what it feels like because that is what it is. My heart, bird-broken, starts to heal its rends. To lay them side by side upon my chest is the first pure right in almost a fortnight of dislocated wrongs. I hadn't even known that this was possible. I hadn't known to ask.

And then the babies begin to squeak. It sounds as if I have a shoebox of baby mice – not quite in canon, but they squeak with deliberation. It is not a noise I've heard from either child before. Squeak. Squeak. Squeak. Squeak. Luciana begins gesturing frantically to Raakhi but before Raakhi can cross the room to listen they have gone quiet and both girls are asleep, instantly and deeply, as if someone had switched them off. They have inched together and are touching lightly, forehead to forehead. Slowly their faces turn, until they are breathing not only supplemental oxygen but each other's warm breath. Luciana points in silence at their monitors. Their blood pressure has stabilised. Their pulses are calm and steady, beating in perfect time.

*

This is how I dreamed first touch would be: the world's new shocking chill slipped into and out of within seconds; an icy plunge before a return to heat and safety on a mother's chest. This is home now, another apartment perhaps, but in the same building as before, its familiar scent one of comfort, its soundtrack the same but louder now, and clearer, unmuffled by viscous fluids and walls of thick taut muscle. Two beings can never come closer than when one entirely encloses the other, wholly dependent, and at birth the baby must become a being apart. But she is in another way drawn nearer: face to face, finally, with a once-inhabited being.

Her mother strokes her hair, her face, her eyelids, her lips, she kisses the new brow. This touch is characteristic, ritualistic, animal and ancient. Another mammal might lick its offspring clean to strip it of the dangerous signs of newness, of vulnerability, but we humans touch with fingertips and also with our language – *My baby*, says the mother, telling the baby who she is. *My baby. Hello, darling.* Baptised by her mother's tears, the healthy newborn isn't crying now; she is calm, and within her is a plastic, immature nervous system codifying the pleasure of deliberate touch, of deliberate tenderness. *Ah, yes.* From touch comes pleasure, from touch comes closeness and deep healing sleep, and nourishment.

What did my daughters first learn of touch?

From their notes I learn that intubation was *attempted but unsuccessful* – these notes do not elaborate on the duration of this assault, nor what the children suffered as gloved hands forced a tube down their constricting throats. Then, *I can't bloody get it in, let's try CPAP*, and the mask and prongs clamped tightly over nose and mouth. Hands and feet bent and flexed with functional dispassionate care, turned this way and that in the white light to find a vein. New, deliberate, focused, startling pain with the introduction of a needle and, through all of this, there was exposure, flailing terror and confusion, the opposite of all known containment.

All done to save them. But through it all I could not even offer them my voice because I wasn't there. Now I can try but on it goes – heels pricked and squeezed like lemons for scant drops of blood, palpation and examination, the scans and procedures and cannulas, the medicalised touch far more frequent than the supervised compensating tenderness that Gabe and I are permitted. There cannot but be costs to these beginnings, impossible to quantify them yet or maybe ever. And now, tonight, the two girls will be parted and we can be with each of them precisely half as often.

*

In the middle of the ward is a heavy-duty black and yellow stretcher, adult-sized, which looks as if it has been made for a building site. Strapped on top is what can only be described as a submarine, or perhaps a one-baby rocket ship. It is about three feet long, and bullet-shaped, as if someone is going to load it into a giant hydraulic tube at a bank and send it shooting up through the ceiling. The bottom half is royal blue fibreglass. The top half is Perspex, with hatches that open to admit a single miniature astronaut, and smaller portholes for ministering to her, mid-flight. The nurses set about interior decorating this pod. A long sausage of muslins arranged in a U-shape, over which is laid another one to create a hammock. Then together, two of them lift B-lette, one holding the baby, the other holding together her thick rope of wires and cables. Once she is positioned, another muslin, printed with elephants, is tucked up to her chin. A portable monitor the size of a transistor radio is connected and balanced at the head end of the stretcher. The nurse briefs the ambulance crew even though she, too, will accompany B-lette on her journey. One baby, three adults and an ambulance. It looks very cosy. It looks utterly petrifying.

Where's the rest of her kit? asks one of the paramedics, and I realise he is asking not about medical devices but her possessions. This seems a gravely respectful acknow-ledgement of her personhood. In actual fact, B-lette has accumulated quite a few belongings. She has her Zaky hand. She has her dummy. She has her memory box, which the nurses dutifully packed up on the trolley beside her pod, even though I attempted to abandon it here. She has a pink laminated teddy bear sign on which is printed her full name – SEGAL Female/Infant TWO – and her birth weight – 1175g. She has a few nappies, a bag of cotton wool and her own pot of Sudocrem. She has a spare hat.

B-lette is wide awake. A bare arm snakes up from beneath the covers and begins to wave. *Not waving but drowning* comes instantly to mind but in fact she doesn't seem distressed, she is merely staring, black-eyed, at the unaccustomed open air above her. The transfer nurse captures the rogue hand and tucks it back in, and the roof is latched shut like a treasure chest. In her pod B-lette is smooth and neat as a bean. Through the clear roof of her rocket she stares up, unblinking. Brave little astronaut. Off she goes on her solo mission, launched into space. There are too many bodies and I am not allowed to go in the ambulance.

Her incubator is wheeled away to be cleaned for its next occupant, leaving only empty floor. I stand fixed upon this ground as if it is hallowed, and wonder, will A-lette realise, when she wakes, that she is alone?

*

The hospital in which my children were born was only completed recently and this space, with its broad flanks of steel and glass, was erected to care for women and their children. The floors of the new Central Hospital are given over entirely to Reproductive Health, Maternal and Fetal Medicine, Women's Cancer and Neonatology. Whatever scenes of gore might take place on its wards and in its theatres, whatever existential battles, the public spaces of the building are the picture of cleanliness and calm, of encouraging posters in pastel shades depicting neatly pregnant women sitting demurely on Swiss balls. It is an NHS facility with the hallways and elevators of private practice. Most of the patients passing in and out of the sliding doors appear to be healthy women in various stages of high- or low-risk pregnancy. Lives begin and end in this building every day, but from the tranquil foyer you would never know it.

At our new home at the Local, it feels as if lives might begin and particularly end in the foyer itself. It is high Victorian, in architecture and atmosphere. Here are returned to the mass of humanity, to broken limbs and acute appendicitis, drunken head lacerations and contagion. Here is paediatric outpatients, where toddlers protest upcoming vaccinations and schoolchildren snap gum, and race up and down on wheeled sneakers. Here is chemotherapy and radiology, here are clattering stretchers, rattling IV poles, buggies packed with staring children. Down that corridor, thataway, is the permanent revolving telenovela of Accident & Emergency. On the first floor is the vast canteen, the newsagent and the coffee shop, Pastry Place. The creaking lifts are as packed as a rush-hour train. When I arrived this morning an old man in a mustard velour dressing gown was hacking up gobs of green phlegm into a handkerchief, in the closed circulating air of the elevator. Between the second and third floor I turned almost blue with holding my breath. I am glad that he is being taken care of but as soon as I feel able, I resolve to take the stairs. At each turn of the endless linoleum corridors is a dispenser of hand sanitiser and I use them all, reaching for the lever even before the last squirt has dried.

One is constantly reminded that this is a Victorian building carved up on the principles of function rather than aesthetics; several rooms have a surreal half a window, where a bisecting wall has been thrown up, in almost deliberate defiance of symmetry or beauty. Locked doors, like a secure psychiatric unit. A suspicious buzzing, and an interview through the video monitor, for admission.

Inside the NICU the wards are small and low-ceilinged, with incubators in close enough proximity that an adult standing between two can easily touch both. The room is on the third floor, but feels underground. The lighting scheme might best be described as 'university nightclub' – little beyond the purpling jaundice lamps and the tiny flashing green and red bulbs of an ear-shaped noise monitor. Intensive Care has a single large window at the back, which reveals not the outside world but a small isolation room, which will be our new home. On a routine test before she moved here, it was discovered that B-lette carries a bug called ceftazidime-resistant pseudomonas. She herself is asymptomatic, but has become a danger to others. In the same breath I am told both that it can be deadly and to forget all about it. Happily! I have enough worries that I am not permitted to set aside.

Immediately opposite our private suite (clever B-lette, with her sinister, dormant bug) is the expressing room. It is long, like a corridor, and has a row of low green chairs against the wall, each separated into its own individual cubicle by floor-length hospital curtains. At one end is a kitchen sink with a stainless-steel draining board, a white bottle of antiviral washing-up liquid and a stack of paper hand towels, swelling with damp. On the shelves above this sink are hand-outs from long-ago lactation workshops, and a collection of very large, very round knitted breasts, of varying ethnicities, stacked into a pyramid like oranges at a greengrocer's.

Expressing alone in my little changing room, with the click-clack of the pump, the drip of the milk is turned to something shameful by its concealment. I succumb instantly and immediately to the hopeless giving-up of the unobserved. I eat a salad with my fingers. I drop crumbs all over myself from a Pea Protein Cookie, my mother's latest odd, restorative delivery. I believe I am alone in here, but behind a curtain it is hard to tell. I fight the urge to race back to the Central Hospital where, for now, I still have an equal right to be. From now on, wherever I am there will be somewhere, vital, urgent, that I am not.

*

Kemisha is in the milking shed in the Central Hospital when later that evening I fall through the door like a storm-swept traveller into the warmth of a friendly tavern. She is reading a magazine while she pumps, picking delicately through a packet of Haribo. I want to lay my head in her lap.

It's shit there, I report, ashamed at the break in my voice. I am homesick for this place, to which I wish I had never had to come.

Kemisha sets down her magazine. *Why did you let them take her? How are you meant to be in two places at once?*

I shrug, helplessly, unwrapping one of the sterile pump kits that will soon be a long-lost luxury. It has not yet been two hours since I expressed at the Local but they will need milk here too, before I leave for the night. Amongst various uncertainties, my body's ability to keep up with this redoubled schedule is not a foregone conclusion.

I have absolutely no idea how to answer Kemisha. I was given no choice in the matter, yet somehow I know that she would never have found herself in this position. She is not told, but consulted.

Already these last days it feels as if I can never give enough of myself to two babies; while I am holding one, the other is without me. One twin must always be waiting. Sophie often sings soft serenades to William, tender lullabies blown like kisses through a porthole to a son who at present is once again too sick to be held. I must pretend not to hear.

But I do hear, we hear each other, and from Sophie I learned to wrap my babies in my voice. Now I talk and sing relentlessly, not only to the daughter on my chest but in the hopes that my other child, enclosed in her Tupperware, can at least sense that I'm near. Unacknowledged, Sophie and I catch songs from one another. Now I must waste hours travelling back and forth, with neither girl, and if I want to see the doctors on both ward rounds I must move fast every morning. My current speed is ponderous, at best. Being in two places at once: yet another requirement fallen into the centre of a newly-described Venn diagram, the overlapping states of the impossible and the necessary.

Anne Lamott writes that when you are in difficulty *your friends surround you like white blood cells.* That is what the women of the milking shed are, I think. We are a massed immune reaction, rising up to battle after injury. We are each other's natural killer cells; it is both an instinct and a deliberate choice of these women to be strong for one another in this wounded women's space. Kemisha offers me a gummy snake, and I take two. Distracted, I turn the pump up too high and yelp.

Hey, honey. Kemisha sets her bottle of milk into one of the cup-holders on top of the mint-green pump, and clips up her bra. *Here. Give me your phone, let's get a WhatsApp group sorted before you have to leave.*

Into my head drifts the phrase, *It takes a village to raise a child.* We as a culture have lost that village. In need, the women of the milking shed have built one.

DAY TWELVE

Wednesday, 14th October

Glory be. The transfer nurse rang this morning to say that there is another bed at the Local and so, shortly after lunch, A-lette will be on the move. A-lette and B-lette, Tom and Jerry, double trouble back together. I know the drill now. Skip a feed, extra caffeine, a touch of extra oxygen and then the submarine will surface for her and she will be loaded into her pod, Navy SEAL on a brave solo mission.

Gabe is at home, going quietly insane in the exile of his sore throat. He is primarily worried about me, martyring my way back and forth. He might have a point; standing up on a lurching Tube train makes me feel as if my wound might rupture with grenade-force, spilling my intestines on to the carriage floor.

Everyone is desperate to give me lifts. Wild to help, my sister has virtually sewn herself a chauffeur's cap. I long for the normality and comfort of seeing her, but the traffic is abysmal and I do not have time to waste, inching up and down through a congested city. The train takes a brief and brutal sixteen minutes. Also I cannot talk to other humans from the outside world, even my most beloved humans. I learned yesterday that moving between hospitals I feel strung out to the point of madness; leaving one and simultaneously approaching the other makes me slightly short-circuit. Seconds count, during these purgatorial journeys. All my energies must be concentrated upon making the train go faster with the power of my will.

So today – first to the Local, where ward round happens an hour earlier. When I arrive B-lette is sleeping, an arm thrown rather casually over her face like a sunbather shielding her eyes. Her 'cares' have already been performed and she will soon be woken by the ward round examination, so I cannot disturb her. I retreat to the uninspiring expressing corridor and update Gabe. *All good at the Local. B-lette asleep. Room still shit.*

But my first ward round is a whole different animal. The consultant, Deepak, is warm and avuncular. There is no indication that parents are the greatest impediment to the practice of his medicine. He makes a great many jokes about the superficial state of this hospital, which is generous as it means I do not need to disguise my anxiety, which remains on red alert. There is an awareness that the initial impression is somewhat ... scrappy. *They are very flashy*, he says, *those big shots over there. But you will see. We can hold our own and what's more, we have heart.* I have heard this line before but from Deepak I believe it.

Deepak gives B-lette a careful once-over. When he first opens her incubator he says, *Nice to meet you, darling. My name is Deepak and I am going to be your consultant*, and I decide that I love this man, readily and completely. How much harder must this work be, how much higher the stakes, acknowledging the infant's humanity; the necessary suffering inflicted by healing hands. I hope B-lette can understand his pronounced Indian accent. *Sorry, darling*, he keeps saying, *sorry, darling, oh, you aren't going to like this one bit, but you can go back to sleep in one more minute. Well done.* He seems roundly pleased by his findings and lavishes praise upon her. Her colour is excellent, she took yesterday's transfer in her stride, she has settled in beautifully. I am given the impression she is a prodigy, unprecedented, an extraordinarily advanced pre-term infant. Papers may be written. I bask in her brilliance. *See, we are ready for the whole family.* Deepak gestures to the empty bay beside B-lette. It hurts a little less to leave her in Deepak's care, knowing that later today he will take charge of both girls. A pressure eases in my chest. I set off into town, for the final time.

By 10 a.m. I am back at the Central Hospital, where there is a new sign on the door announcing a local chicken pox outbreak, and the consequent suspension of even the most limited remaining visiting rights. Only parents, under any circumstances. Today I have a totally new attitude. *Let's get the hell out of here, then. Let's get this show on the road.*

A-lette is asleep, cool as a cucumber, and so I sit beside her and listen to the bustle of the moving malarkey. I am an old hand, now. I am familiar with the pre-move comings and goings, the brandishing of paperwork, the transfer nurse appearing and disappearing, the signing and conferring and planning. It is a delicate operation with many moving parts – two hospitals, two transfer coordinators, the ambulance team and the labour ward, who might well make decisions about a mid-level emergency based on the availability of an incubator.

Our departure will make way for someone else from another room or another hospital or perhaps someone as yet unborn, whose birth can now be scheduled. It is odd to think we may occasion someone's birthday.

I am calm, but A-lette seems to be feeling the pressure. The alarms from her incubator are going off with increasing regularity, and insistence. These are not her usual dips but deeper, longer, more frequent. The monitor shows her oxygen levels falling lower and lower, and staying down for longer troughs. 85%. 82%. 79%. 70%. After a morning cruising around 98%, now she needs her supplemental oxygen cranked higher and higher just to keep her sitting into the low nineties. After the second of these adjustments the nurse frowns into her incubator. *What are you playing at, young lady?* she says. *We'll have no silly buggers today, thank you very much.*

Something is going wrong. *Her colour's off*, the nurse says, and I look at her, helplessly. I am rarely able to discern these changes that they see so readily – to me, their skin always looks mottled, fragile, painfully translucent. The baby is grunting now, and wheezing. A junior doctor pops her head round the door, but the nurse ignores her and pages the consultant.

A-lette's heart rate keeps dropping, and each time seems less and less able to recover. Her intercostal muscles are recessing with the effort to breathe. Now, even I can tell that her colour is all wrong. She looks mottled and pallid and flushed, at the same time.

And then all her alarms are wailing. She has stopped breathing, and does not seem able or willing to start again. The nurse shakes her, not very gently, and rubs her chest. *Come on, you naughty girl*, she whispers, *stop messing with us.*

Suddenly, the swing doors are pushed open and the room is filled with bottle green – the ambulance crew has arrived. They are pushing a stretcher, on which is the bright blue submarine pod, ready to whisk A-lette to her sister's side.

Who's ready to hit the road? asks the taller medic, brightly.

No one in this room, says the nurse under her breath. Her hand is still on my daughter's now heaving chest. On the monitor the numbers are correcting. *Hold your horses*, she tells him.

Harriet, the consultant, arrives, taking in the green uniforms, the stretcher, the space pod. She listens to the nurse recount the details of the last half-hour.

Start her on ceftazidime and teicoplanin, take a screen. She needs a chest X-ray. I don't think her anaemia is helping the breathing, I'll write her up for a blood transfusion. To me she says, *I think she has an infection from the longline removal yesterday. We're starting intravenous antibiotics.*

Then she turns to the ambulance drivers. These are not the same as yesterday's crew; still, they have a jolly familiarity, a sturdy competence. Their uniform, the badges and boots, the wide-legged stance, all faintly armed forces. They stand with their hands folded behind their backs in silent attendance.

I am really sorry about this, but she's not fit to travel. They nod. There is no protest; they simply begin to pack away the kit, the mobile monitors, the leads and wires. Harriet turns back to me. *You understand I have to do this. It wouldn't be safe. She doesn't seem very well.*

It is hours later when I take my phone from my pocket to see a series of messages from Gabe. *Are you there? How was transfer? Did they let you ride with her? How are you? Don't forget to have lunch!*

*

Harriet comes back to check on A-lette. We've been waiting for the results of the blood tests to come, but there is still no sign of them and she can't tell me how much longer it will be. A-lette is a sick little girl, but no one yet knows why. But they will need milk, soon, at the other hospital, and if I don't leave in the next hour I will not have very long there before I am kicked out for handover. Harriet tells me to go. *We'll phone you if we get news.* I suppose handover will be a good time to travel back in the other direction, again.

I left B-lette this morning, thriving and cosy in her new digs. But when I get to her bedside at the Local I learn that she too has had an eventful time of it. She has needed more and more oxygen throughout the day, and her colour was off. The nurse summons Deepak who decides to run another cannula and put B-lette on the same cocktail of intravenous antibiotics as her sister. Not a line infection, then, but something contagious. They were reunited on my chest only yesterday, and shared more than they should.

At handover, I stagger back to the Central Hospital. I cry openly as I negotiate the stairs down into the station; there is something reassuring about the knowledge that on a busy evening commute it is likely no one will ask me if I am okay, nor offer to help. Instead, everyone steps carefully or not so carefully around me. Rain evaporates from the crush of winter coats and in the humid carriage I hold the rail above my head with one hand and hold on to myself very tightly with the other, clutching my stomach like a bad actress. A man leaps up to give me his seat. I start rather madly to say, *No, no, it's all right*, but then fall into it and double over, my face on my knees, which feels much better. The corset of pain begins to loosen. The station I'm heading for has escalators, so that is better, too. I wonder if there are more or stronger drugs I can take, but probably not, or surely they would have given them to me. There is a battle currently raging within my daughters and I wonder what will win, the bacteria or the antibiotics. I wonder if it is in fact a virus. If it is Gabe's cold, I only hope he never knows it. I wonder if they miss each other.

DAY THIRTEEN

Thursday, 15th October

Gabe drank five litres of water and took a rock star's overdose of Vitamin C yesterday, and is no longer a biohazard. So he went to A-lette at the Central Hospital while I came to the Local, and B-lette. Both babies are rallying; the magical antibiotics appear to be winning.

B-lette is asleep on her side. Her oxygen is still higher than it has been for days, but she's had a stable night. In one of my palms a foot; in the other I hold her head, peach-sized, peach fuzzed with pale hair, and in this way I try to contain her as best I can, with firm, static pressure.

My hands are impossibly close together, yet between them is a human child. I clenched them for a long time beneath a scalding tap before touching her, to take away their natural chill. Today she weighs 1.190kgs.

I am already devoted to everyone at our new hospital. I have love-heart eyes, gazing around at them all. I understand now what the nurses were trying to explain before this move. The pace of a Level Two unit is so different, the atmosphere is calmer, the same alarms sound, but less frequently – and they're usually not the other babies, but mine. Everything is relative, and it is we who are the troublemakers here.

From isolation, the window into the main ward opens to us like a theatre. It is as if we are behind a one-way mirror, watching the action within. You cannot hear through the glass but often nurses signal to one another, with hand gestures and waves. Today three monstrously large full-term babies lie in a row beneath strong jaundice lamps, lit as blue as a tanning shop. Closer to our window are two babies born overnight, creatures of such startlingly different appearance from each other that I hadn't known they were twins until Deepak told me. In the far corner is a hearty boy with a full head of black hair and frowning black brows. He has a feeding tube but is breathing alone, and when I walked past this morning was crying lustily, with the lung capacity of a bagpiper. In the next incubator is a tiny, hirsute little scrap, in CPAP hat and hose, less than half the size. They had Twin-to-Twin Transfusion Syndrome, in which identical twins sharing a placenta get uneven slices of the pie. Their time *in utero* was worthy of an opera: two brothers, one living high off the hog; one starving like a pauper. I cannot help my own slight feelings of outrage at the selfishness of the fatter one.

I am sitting very still. Within the incubator, my hands are occupied; the rest of me, most notably my mind, has nothing to do. It has never been my way but I must learn how to simply *be*. Then in my back pocket my phone vibrates.

Hang out the bunting! A-lette is on the move. Have you left anything in the locker?

I think for a minute. *A grapefruit.*

Bit rushed here, but looks like they're going to let me ride in ambulance with her. I wonder what it says about Gabe's impression of my state of mind when a moment later he adds, *But would you like me to go back and get it?*

DAY FOURTEEN

Friday, 16th October

Winter is approaching. It is pale grey when I get up to come in; it is thick night-darkness by the time I go home. Soon the clocks will go back for Daylight Saving and the last dusky light will have faded by late afternoon, but to us it makes little difference. The nurses discuss the curse of that upcoming shift with theatrical shivers of horror – whoever's on must work an extra hour, that night. I have not been outside in daylight for two weeks.

Nothing has come back on any of the cultures, and if A-lette and B-lette get one more clean set of blood tests we can stop their antibiotics. A double reprieve.

Deepak says their slump was probably The Slump. The first days of life are honeymoon days, a false proficiency, beginner's luck at the all-consuming novelty of independent homeostasis. But eventually comes depletion of the very little iron and energy reserves accrued *in utero*, and then comes exhaustion, and a crash. *I can do this,* the babies seem to say in disbelief, *but you never said you expected me to keep doing it for ever*.

Poor babies. Living is hard bloody work.

DAY FIFTEEN

Saturday, 17th October

I keep calling upon Sophie for help with the naming situation. It's possible I am driving her mad, though she appears to take it well. I don't know – this is all conducted by text, from my hospital to hers. Still. What else do we have to do all day?

Olympia.

She'd be Olly.

Lilith.

Flawless feminist credentials. Uptight wife in Frasier still a problem?

Cecily.

What if she has a lithp?

Genuinely quite attached to A-lette and B-lette.

A-lette and William invite you to their wedding ...

BTW, on that subject, I was not into the Martin situation. The day we left, Sunny's mother tried to get in on the action by suggesting, via Sunny, that B-lette and Martin were the obvious next betrothal in Nursery One. *He's perfectly eligible, but I am not pumping all this breast milk only for my daughter to bugger off to Korea. Lucky we ran away to the Local when we did. #Awkward!*

Completely. If we ever actually get William breastfeeding I am never going to stop. Hope A-lette won't mind. I'll be discreet. Stay out of the way on honeymoon etc.

Frederica?

Love AS Byatt, she replies, *V. Strong. Frederica and what? Doesn't really go with B-lette.*

Thomasina? From Arcadia.

I mean, embrace the pretension, I say. Freddy and Tommy?

Hadn't thought but of course. Cute unless they're built like tanks?

Teeny tiny little micro-tanks.

DAY SIXTEEN

Sunday, 18th October

For the first time there was another mother in the parents'
kitchen this morning when I went in to refill my water bottle.
She was in a baggy Arsenal jumper, her hair waxed back into
a high, tight ponytail with the sort of large hoop earrings that
would be a provocation for any real babies – captivating
shiny rings for little hands to grab. She was leaving as I arrived
and so I stopped in the doorway with a slightly desperate
smile. *Hi*, I said brightly, extending my hand. *I'm Francesca.*

She gave the hand a long look. *Izzit*, she said. I stepped
aside quickly as she shouldered past.

Day Sixteen

All round, today has been a spectacular exercise in futility. Neither girl has woken since I arrived and 'DESATS ON HANDLING' is scrawled all over both their notes, which means the oxygen level in their blood falls whenever they are touched. The nurses are not unduly worried; it is just that the babies seem to want to be alone with their own thoughts this morning. As a writer I should recognise this instinct, still I am mildly affronted. They have become teenagers, apparently, and I am advised to give them their personal space. I could have spent the last six hours in bed, or working, or drinking champagne in a hot tub, for all they would have noticed.

At the Central Hospital I would retreat to the milking shed where this precise sensation of trapped and urgent uselessness is taken for granted. It would take so little shorthand to be completely understood there. *They can't come out* would be enough for someone to curse in sympathy, for someone else to make a bad joke, or offer me a Hobnob. Instead, I steel myself to go back in to isolation. I find this kitchen unspeakably depressing, with its low, mourners' seats, its basket of ratty toys for visiting siblings. If a baby is dying on the ward, this room is requisitioned for her parents to stay, and so to leave space for the opened sofa bed there is no coffee table. One must clutch one's mug on one's knees like someone in the shock of recent bad news. And at least on the ward I am on hand if either baby deigns to stir and summon me.

As I heave myself up, my phone beeps.

Yo. Where's good for coffee near your gaff?

Sophie and William are in an ambulance, on their way to the Local. Hallelujah.

DAY SEVENTEEN

Monday, 19th October

Oh, Mummy. I'm glad you're here. It is Perlah, a nurse I love, extending indigo-gloved hands to me. *Twin One – your A-lette – has not been very happy. Oh, Mummy,* she says again, and the pity in her eyes stops my breath. *It is so good you are here.*

You could have called in the night, I start to say, moving towards the incubator as if underwater, *I would have come,* but it turns out this has just happened; is still happening, things began to go wrong at 5 a.m. and the registrar was bleeped before six; a new cannula delivering a triple-strength cocktail of antibiotics has only just been sited in a new place, high up, above a previous entry point on her right foot, still unhealed. Perlah was on her way to phone us when I walked through the door. Everything points to the same thing: Necrotising Enterocolitis. The doctors believe that part of A-lette's bowel is dying.

Perlah has positioned the baby on her back, ribs splaying, her heart fluttering with the shallow speed of a trapped sparrow's. A-lette is struggling to catch her breath. In a matter of hours she has taken on the shape of famine: domed, distended belly. Her mouth is open; her forehead is creased with deep furrows. She is suffering. At thirty-three weeks gestational age she cannot know her own boundaries but pain teaches, and today it blooms within the right side of her abdomen like a lily unfolding, expanding and sharpening her definition of her self. *There, yes, just there, that hurts, that is within me.*

My biggest little girl. I have watched the shadows of dreams pass across her face, her eyelids flutter in who-knows-what remembered arcs and leaps and cartwheels. I cannot guess what she recalls, nor what she may conjecture. The seventeen days since her birth have been a confused assault of disorganised associative learning; the model she must be constructing is of life as suffering and solitude, deliberately inflicted. In it she is almost entirely without agency, or temporal anchor. Now the in-out-in-out of breathing is all consuming, but she does not know why she must fight, nor whether the fight will end.

My instinct is deep, and primitive: I want to curl myself around her like a force field; I want to shield her with my body as if from an earthquake. I want to snatch her up and retreat alone to the back of a cave like an animal. But when her need is greatest, I am not allowed to hold her. All I can do instead is wash my hands again, open her porthole, and offer up my softest voice, and hope that it will wind into her dreams and there comfort her. I lay my arm across the bottom of her nest so that the raw pink soles of her feet rest against the inside of my wrist. This is the most contact she can tolerate, and the least that I can stand. The last hours have been bad ones. And I, her mother, have not been there.

Sophie: *V. odd goldfish bowl set up in this place. Decided not to be English and pretend I couldn't see you in your tank over there. You don't look great, F. Everything alright?*

Me: *Not really. A-lette has NEC.*

We are probably only twenty feet apart, but there is a wall of sound-proof glass between us. I look up and Sophie gives a bleak smile. She knows the prognosis, just as I do. In babies under 1500g, like ours, Necrotising Enterocolitis has a survival rate below 50 per cent.

Sophie: *I'm sorry. Shit. Fuck.*

Yes. Fuck, I text back.

*

Above where we sit are two screens side by side, B-lette's steady rhythmic waves and A-lette's increasing struggle translated into erratic graphs. Her alarms sound over and over.

We wait together for her sister's ultrasound, B-lette and I. Gabe is coming from work as fast as he can, but he was almost an hour away. In the meantime I choose to think about names. I want to draw B-lette into the discussion but, perhaps to conceal her anxiety for her sister, B-lette sleeps on and on, so I muse aloud only to myself. Freddy and Tommy. *Hello, little person*, I try. *Is your name by any chance Frederica? How would you like to be Thomasina?* Sophie is right, the names may be alike, but the characters they evoke are worlds apart. Byatt's Frederica is messier, more abrasive, more complicated, far less 'likeable', in contemporary parlance – but she has the more depth for it.

She gets second and third chances. She comes to motherhood, and a circuitous, satisfying career. She reaches maturity, and lives long enough to risk imperfection. Frederica Potter inhales and grasps and lives. Killed in a house fire on the eve of her seventeenth birthday, Stoppard's sweet Thomasina Coverly is merely the shaded promise of a woman. No, despite the shared cadence, despite the shared evocation of masculinity feminised, the names are not equals. In any case, my daughters do not need to solve Fermat's Last Theorem, nor go to Cambridge, nor widely dazzle. They need only to live.

If we lose a daughter, what stories will remain? What will I be able to give B-lette of the sister she once had? *She was fractionally bigger than you. The bow of her lips had a slightly different arc.* I have so little of them still, they are barely differentiated. Inside each tiny teacup skull a private world of brief experience and sensation, of vivid baby-thought, but I have known none of it.

No Thomasinas here, I tell sleeping B-lette, *no thank you.* We need names for grown women. For mothers. For healthy, hearty grandmothers. But already I know we have come too far, that Gabe and I will not be able to choose their names until we know which way this will go.

*

A-lette's ultrasound is over, and Deepak doesn't think it's NEC.

Well, darling, he said, ever courtly, addressing his findings almost entirely to A-lette, *whatever is going on with you is not good, but it is less not good than we thought. All the action is taking place in your duodenum, which is a very long word, darling, du-o-de-num. Forget all about it. But it is very high in your gut, and usually NEC is lower down. Let us not even talk about NEC any more, in fact.* This last quite firm, as if it had been she, the baby, harping on obsessionally about it and at last Deepak was putting his foot down.

Deepak turned from A-lette to me and Gabe. *It isn't NEC. And she is responding beautifully to the antibiotics. It is possible we will never know exactly what this was, but in some ways –* he raises his palms – *whatever it is, she is getting better. What can I say? They like to keep us on our toes, these babies.*

Meanwhile, tiny B-lette is in fine fettle, saturating perfectly throughout the afternoon – she has seen off The Slump with aplomb. The upside of this for B-lette is that Gabe and I have performed a new manoeuvre, and for the first time we have passed a baby one to the other. When

Gabe arrived I had been holding her for hours and, having given up on the naming exercise, was reading aloud to her from Twitter. As a form of procrastination she seemed to like it; perhaps she will become a journalist. But after a while I was numb from thigh to coccyx, desperately needing the loo, and so I asked the nurse if we might swap. She lifted B-lette up, I slipped out, and Gabe slid in in my place. B-lette was plopped back down, unfussed. As it stands she has had a seven-hour cuddle today. I was all set to swap back in again after the success of the first time, but then it was handover and we had to leave.

Not NEC. Another reprieve. Another stroke of luck. I do not, not for one moment, take it for granted.

*

It's night-time on the ward, when we come back. The lights are low in isolation. B-lette's incubator is muffled beneath its quilted cover and within she lies in darkness, sleeping off her marathon adventure. But A-lette's is flipped back, and Jamila is talking to her softly, through the porthole. Jamila looks up when we come in.

We've got a very hungry baby, here.

A-lette is crying, a thin animal mew. Intravenous dextrose is about as satisfying to her as it sounds to us. Jamila returns her gaze to the baby.

You are not very impressed with us this evening, are you? I wouldn't have thought her up to coming out but it's not good for her to be so agitated, either. Let's see if a cuddle with Mummy can calm you down.

I hadn't expected A-lette to be well enough for days. I all but tear open my shirt and Jamila sets the baby high upon my chest and instantly I can breathe. Tears run in a steady stream down the sides of my face but I stay completely silent, completely still. She needs me calm and so I choose to release the horror of the day, and let it drift from me. But A-lette has other ideas. Far from settling, she is frantic now. Her head lurches from side to side, her mouth is working, her cries redoubled. It is as if the hunger has awoken her instincts. She knows what I am for now.

Jamila looks down at her. *Well, there's no mistaking what you want, missy.* She asks when I last expressed, and I tell her I have just now come from the pump. *Poor darling, it's not good for her to be so upset. Let's get her to try.*

Jamila pushes us towards one another as if we are two shy children told to play. The pressure of Jamila's hand upon mine is far harder than I would have expected and the stiff, angry baby latches on and softens, melting into my arms. She sucks as though she's always known it, only pausing after a moment to release a small, mouse-squeak of a sigh. The tender warmth of her mouth is as far from the unyielding brutality of the pump as I can imagine, and she is so small that my two hands touch as I hold her. I cannot take my eyes from the miracle that she is.

This moment feels transgressive; it feels sacred; and I realise that Jamila has restored to us a stolen intimacy, has swept away an alienation I hadn't even known lay between me and my daughters. I am feeding my baby. I have always been feeding her, in fact, and the infant knows it, and she knows me. I have felt myself taken from them so completely that I could not trust that my children recognised their mother, until now. How could I know?

This morning I thought my daughter was dying. For a time, I believe that she was, until alert and tireless medics laid down new track: benzylpenicillin, gentamicin, metronidazole, and upon these blessed rails her train could run a different course. Now we have arrived here. Tonight, for the first time, she lies in my arms and at my breast, like a baby. And I recognise in my own shape – the length of my bowed neck, the fall of my hair as I gaze down at my nursing infant – that my body is the shape of a mother.

DAY EIGHTEEN

Tuesday, 20th October

Sophie: *Morning ladies, who's up and milking? Or for that matter, dancing up a storm in a dirty club/writing poetry by candlelight in fingerless gloves/having a threesome etc.*

Me: *I'm up. Having a threesome with a DJ I picked up in a dirty club and a poet in fingerless gloves, how did you guess?*

Kemisha: *:) HAHA. I'm here 2.*

Sophie: *How was today for everyone?*

Kemisha: *2day pretty good. Evanee breastfed for 15 minutes!*

Sophie: *Wooohoo! Go Evanee!*

Me: *That's our girl!*

Sophie: *And well done Evanee's mummy.*

Kemisha: *Yeah but then she slept for like 18hrs & we tube fed, she was knackered.*

Sophie: *She'll get there. It's hard work, sucking. I wouldn't be bothered if I was them.*

Me: *I sometimes think I'd quite like an NG tube, so someone could feed me while I slept …*

Sophie: *I know, no wonder they're so attached to them, we're spoiling them with convenience. Why buy the boob when you can get the milk for free?*

Kemisha: *How's ur crew, F? U had crazy day, yesterday.*

Me: *B-lette good. A-lette on the mend I think, but cannula keeps leaking, they had to move it again. It's a million times a day at the moment. We're running out of limbs.*

Sophie: *:-O Poor little pincushion.*

Kemisha: *Don't let junior doc do next 1! Ask 4 consultant.*

Me: *Can we do that??!*

Kemisha: *I do! My baby ain't a training dummy.*

Sophie: *K, can you come to my next ward round and tell them to try William on Optiflow, please? Actually, can you come to all my ward rounds?*

Kemisha: *;)*

Me: *K, you should run assertiveness workshops.*

Sophie: *Duh, she's already running assertiveness workshops right here, you've been enrolled for weeks. Not K's fault we are slow learners …*

Kemisha: *U girls, hahaha. I'll get u there eventually.*

DAY NINETEEN

Wednesday, 21st October

A-lette's cannula site is red and so the line in her wrist has to come out yet again. Anton is coming to put it back again, wonderful Anton who is one of the doctors we love, and who is tender and human and approachable.

By now, nineteen days in, I feel myself an odd kind of subsidiary or indentured staff member, no longer a bystander but instead expected to participate at such times as my presence might be useful. I am not ushered from the room during difficult procedures but instead am required to remain and provide reassurance, palliation, restraint. When

Anton inserts his hair-fine needle it will be my hands pinning down my daughter, the scent of my skin in her nostrils. This is supposed to provide familiarity but each time I am complicit in an assault I wonder – is it reassurance I provide, or are we forming a Pavlovian association with pain? Should I instead be stepping aside, absenting myself from her lowest moments, leaving Anton as the villain? I could return, the heroine, to comfort her.

But the staff expect us to comply, and I am still craven in my need for approval. I want to be chosen as head girl, to be praised, to be liked. I want admiration for my commitment and my cleverness. Most of all, I want with my unprecedented brilliance to transcend my children's anonymity. I want us to be visible, to be *seen* by these hard-working doctors who must, with functional self-preserving detachment, minister to an endless parade of patients. I want them to care, so that my children matter.

So. Here is Anton, and here is Anton's needle failing, repeatedly, to find a suitable vein. I am all business, but in a break between attempts I text my friend Adam, deliverer of babies, doctor of happier departments.

How many cannula attempts is a dr allowed before I ask for consultant?

Oh no :-(

A beat.

2x max.

By the time this message reaches me we are long past that. Poor Anton. He is a registrar and he is a good, kind man with gentle, clever hands, a man visibly distressed at the failure of his first try, his second, his third. By the fourth my own hands remain steady unwavering clamps upon his patient but my face is to the sky and silent tears are coursing down my cheeks, an indictment, though I have not spoken. I feel bad for him, planning his intimate wedding in Malmö, working impossibly long shifts, forced to wound for a living the babies he strives to save. I believe he is my age. In another world I think that Anton and I would be friends. Today, though I say nothing, the room vibrates with my sorrow and rage.

Eventually Anton admits defeat and when he withdraws I see that he, too, is close to tears. *Please, Anton*, I say. I try to keep all judgement from my voice. *Get me a Jedi.*

Thomas is the Jedi, Consultant Neonatologist, a stocky, bearded cricketer from Aberystwyth, always good for rugby banter with the nurses who clearly worship him. Thomas explains that every one of my daughter's veins has been broken by previous lines, right hand and left hand, right and left ankle. Anton is vindicated. It was not the workman nor even his tools, but the very clay that was to blame. The new line must be run through her scalp.

Despite everything, that A-lette will need a wet shave feels the evening's greatest act of barbarism. Fine blonde hair falls from the blade like glitter. I press my finger to it, scattered on the giraffe-printed sheets that I laundered this morning, at home. Thomas looks momentarily disturbed. Did I want to keep it, he asks, straight-faced, as if this is not the removal of a near-invisible cap of down but a first curl, tied with ribbon. No doubt he is used to parents making relics of anything and everything – we have so little with which to make memories, here. I shake my head, no, though I know that if he wasn't here, or wasn't watching, I would press my glinting fingertip to my tongue, and swallow.

*

The head cannula is in and, in truth, A-lette cried very little. But it is not stable, the tape doesn't hold it well on the curve of her skull, and babies are renowned for yanking out these particular lines. I see their point. It recalls me to the day the orthodontist tried to convince me to wear my head brace to school. It was one thing to sleep in it, lying rigid as a geisha, but to be seen in public was unthinkable – protruding teeth were better. Why should A-lette be the only kid on the ward to appear in such a humiliating get-up?

As Thomas is speaking, A-lette begins to bash repeatedly at her own forehead, displaying precocious proprioception for a person still many weeks in advance of her own birth, I think, with some pride. But this fighting spirit will have to be subdued. I assume that there is a bit of kit for this but there isn't; this is bush medicine, it seems, and so we have scissors and cotton wool and surgical tape, and we are manufacturing a protective device from the sort of shallow plastic cup in which a nurse might deliver medication. Moments later my child is lying before me with a yogurt pot taped to her gleaming head, affixed at a jaunty angle as though she is dressed, avant-garde, for the Ascot ladies' enclosure. Thomas withdraws, with evident relief to be away from me.

*

On the bus home. The giraffes, clean only this morning, are once again bundled into my bag. I summon up Amazon on my phone. I have always been a Stain Devil devotee – every novelist should keep to hand a bottle of Stain Devil No. 3, for removing ink, biro and crayon. It has rescued me over and over from carelessly dropped pens. Today I am hunting for Stain Devil No. 4 and when I find it, only available from a 'Third-Party Seller', I put six bottles in my basket. It is surprisingly hard to come by these days, though it is an invaluable addition to any laundry cupboard, formulated to tackle the following tough stains, even at low temperatures: red wine, tea, lipstick, mayonnaise, chocolate, ketchup, baby food and blood.

DAY TWENTY

Thursday, 22nd October

On ward round with Deepak this morning, A-lette's headgear drew the crowds. I can't help but notice that it is a different, taller plastic cup, and that the layers of tape have lengthened and multiplied. One piece runs all the way down along her jawline, like a chin strap. The cannula has survived the night but barely, Perlah reports to Deepak, with the baby making ever more devious attempts upon it, and the night nurse forced each time to devise ever more elaborate schemes to fend her off. She needs a cone of the sort vets issue to recalcitrant post-surgical cats. A-lette has put up a spirited resistance and I am jubilant, for just the day before yesterday she was sunk in the lethargy and inward-turn of the gravely ill.

Deepak explains that this turnaround is not unusual – when antibiotics work well then this is how it goes; they can sweep through the body of an infant just as fast as sickness. The exhausting ride of NICU is precisely this – peril and reprieve within hours of one another. I don't know how the staff aren't all stark raving mad with it. Who takes care of these caregivers? What support is there for them, in their indefatigable support of us?

And so A-lette has two problems today: where to site her next cannula, for this one's hours are clearly numbered; and an abdomen that is still uncomfortably bloated. Deepak makes his diagnosis. *Like so many things in life, darling, we have come upon a lesson that you must learn for yourself.* He shakes his head with regret. *You must try. No one else can teach you how to fart.*

When I get home, I find that my mother has made a Moroccan lamb stew with apricot and prunes. On it is a note explaining that the red meat is to address our collective anaemia, mine and the girls; the prunes, she writes, are to help with A-lette's newly diagnosed constipation. Gabe is warned to eat around the prunes. My mother has taken on the task of feeding us with the dedication of a Ph.D. student, and the magical thinking of an Isabel Allende character. In another world, another family, another culture, her love might be expressed as prayer. In ours, my mother's wishes find their expression in recipes. In a time of need she has turned to her God, Jamie Oliver. I think of my own frustrations, my own longing to help and shield A-lette and B-lette, and I almost cannot bear to see myself as I know she must – her child, weighed down by a burden she cannot lift from my shoulders.

I remember in early pregnancy the round ligament pain; the ache as long-stiff parts were stretched, as the body accommodated more and then more within itself. In this way my love for my daughters burgeons and strains against my boundaries; it is greater than the limits of the heart that contains it. It hurts as it burst banks. I cannot understand it, nor what it means for who I am or was. It is relentless and propulsive. It is a dangerous element, this love. It is a risk. I will turn myself inside out. It will flay me.

That my own mother loves me thus I know to be true, have always sensed, and yet to think of it now gives me vertigo. My sorrow at her sorrow in the face of my suffering my daughters' suffering is dizzying. But I watch her turn prayer into eccentric gastronomy and I pass onwards this relay of remote devotions.

Frozen breast milk lasts three months, and so to ensure that the earliest bottles will be used first, I have created a system with the complexity of the Dewey Decimal. Weeks ago I explained this numbering to Gabe with all the stern possessive pride of a librarian orienting a new student, though we both know, or suspect, that I will not allow anyone else to manage these reserves. I now add bottle number 117 (in green Sharpie, not purple, to indicate that it is from home, not hospital), expressed after a midnight supper of Moroccan Prune Tagine, with Lamb. I do not believe this tagine can have agency but, nonetheless, I will upend my own system and feed this new bottle to A-lette tomorrow, in good faith. We open up our selves to one another. We offer up the thought, the wish, the prayer, the laxative by proxy. We each must love as we can. We all must believe in the power of efforts made in love, or our own impotence would drown us.

DAY TWENTY-ONE

Friday, 23rd October

I can't believe you come here without me, Sophie says. We have bumped into one another in the queue at Pastry Place.

I can't believe you *come here without* me. *I introduced you to this place. Quite frankly, you're only somebody around these parts because I put in a good word.*

Sophie sighs. *Sometimes a girl just wants to eat her feelings at,* she looks at her watch, *seven thirty-one a.m., without someone else watching her and thereby inducing further feelings on the subject. You know?*

I get that. Do you want me to also have a chocolate muffin?

That would be chivalrous, yes.

Do you want me to sit at a different table to eat it?

Yes, in fact.

We sit back to back at separate tables, invisible to one another, the legs of our chairs almost touching. Every now and again without turning Sophie will announce a headline from a few pages of yesterday's *Guardian Family* scavenged from another table, and when I receive a text message from my GP's surgery informing me that, as a pregnant woman, I am entitled to a free flu shot, I read this aloud and behind me Sophie snorts with appreciative laughter. At 8 a.m. precisely, when handover will be ending, we each rise and toss our coffee cups and crumpled greaseproof wrappers into the bin and go upstairs, side by side.

DAY TWENTY-TWO

Saturday, 24th October

The tiny wound in A-lette's head from the cannula is healing to a pink freckle. In Phrenology, it lies in the zone of the Reflectives, in what might be Agreeableness and Mirth, or perhaps Causality. Her hairstyle is still somewhat unconventional. I wonder if we should have shaved it all, just for uniformity of regrowth, but I don't know what the nurses would make of it if I asked to do it today. I am always carefully attuned to the possibility of behaving like a nut job. Their psychosocial notes are copious, and closely observed.

A calm day. Gabe and I are here together, reclining beneath matching babies. Behind us the nurses are gossiping quietly. They are not allowed to leave us unattended, but I am grateful for their retreat into their own exchange, for it offers us the closest approximation of privacy. Gabe has A-lette, whose half-reflective head is concealed now beneath a butter-yellow cotton hat. I have B-lette, in a more flamboyant floral number. In moments like these I cannot imagine greater happiness.

Gabe can be my mirror, I his. There is a pleasure in describing them, in claiming them with language for ourselves. *Your one is opening her eyes; she's closing her eyes. She's frowning, she's pursing her lips.* Gabe studies the infant I am holding and says, *That's Celeste.* With my palm I cup her perfect apple head. *Hello, Celeste.*

I look across at the tiny face beneath Gabe's, A-lette, her cheek against her father's chest. I don't think she can see me – today she is three weeks and two days old, still only thirty-three gestational weeks. But I look into her eyes, wide open, monkey-black. *Hello, little person. Do you think that you might be Raffaella?* It is Raffaella who looks back at me steadily. She seems to have no doubt on the subject. Gabe presses his lips to the top of the yellow hat and murmurs, *Hello, Raffaella.*

I think, *Within these names you will grow and shift, they will become the place that you will inhabit.* Raffaella and Celeste. Celeste and Raffaella.

I will miss A-lette and B-lette. Slowly they will recede, layered and folded into the depths of my growing daughters as each becomes herself. *But how lucky we are,* I think madly, feeling this change like a stroke of great fortune, like a glorious accident, *how lucky we are, to have daughters with such beautiful names.*

DAY TWENTY-THREE

Sunday, 25th October

Another full-term baby appears on the main ward, fleetingly, for a brief spell of phototherapy. *Fatty*, Sophie and I text one another, viciously. The mother barely has enough time to stop wailing and rending her collars before her son is discharged back upstairs to his bouquets and teddies and panicked, texting relatives.

'Fatty' is what I've no doubt Sophie thought of my enormous one-kilo babies, born at the same weight that William had been working towards, painstakingly, since August. Darling William. Darling Sophie. Unthinkable to be without them. But if my girls were not a sure thing then William, my future son-in-law, was an odds-defying miracle. I am weak with gratitude that both Sophie and Kemisha have had the grace to forgive me my relative good fortune. I check and am checked by my own privilege among these women. And there it is, restored, my empathy for Fatty's mother, frightened and disoriented by the blue jaundice lights and the unexpected intrusion of the words INTENSIVE CARE into the narrative of her own birth story. Her fear of losing her son was real – I saw it. Why should she be made to place her trauma in rank order? We are all luckier than someone.

DAY TWENTY-FOUR

Monday, 26th October

This afternoon I am finishing off B-lette's feed when a message pings up from Sophie. *This is radical, bear with me.* Through the window I can see a naughty gleam in her eye. *WHAT?* I mouth, with a Jackie Mason shrug. Perlah and Marisol, our respective nurses, smile at one another, two nannies exchanging wry looks about their unexpectedly animated charges. My syringe empties and I detach it, screwing the purple cap back on to the top of B-lette's NG tube. She is sound asleep. I have spent twenty-two minutes feeding her, and the next feed is therefore due in thirty-eight minutes. The rest of Sophie's message arrives. *Shall we go for a walk?*

I give a thumbs-up. *Let's blow this hotdog stand.*

This excursion will not be to eat or sleep. It will simply be for a break, and the pleasure of being with Sophie. I can't bring myself to look down at B-lette, saturating at a heroic 95 per cent, despite the hard toil of digestion. She is curled on her left side, snug beneath the scented weight of her lilac disembodied Muppet hand. This walk will be the first time I have stepped away from her and her sister for anything that wasn't essential. Choosing, briefly but decidedly, to go.

There is no way for me to give A-lette and B-lette the time that most of the other NICU inmates take for granted. While Sophie or Kemisha are here, their sole focus is upon one baby. But whenever I am with one infant, the other is without me. My last few attempts to hold them together have not gone well. One or both has struggled to settle and has found it difficult to breathe, their alarms sounding in protest, and for the moment we have decided to stop trying. There's no obvious reason why it should be so – we all want to believe that nestling them back together will offer the ultimate comfort, but the girls have been extremely clear on the subject. We have not been able to recreate those first magical reunions. I can give my daughters precisely half the hours on my chest, half the feeds, half the touch. I spend double the time of the other women at the breast pump just to keep up, and every day I feel myself losing more and more ground. If I hold one of my daughters for three hours or even four while Gabe holds the other, that still leaves twenty hours she will lie in an incubator, alone.

Sophie is always quite firm when I start on this poor me routine. *You had twins*, she says. *That sense of loyalties divided is how it always would have been for you.* She reminds me of women we knew at the Central Hospital who had no co-parent and two or three or four older children at home quite apart from the one in hospital. These mothers could be on the ward for only a snatched evening, a rushed early-morning visit; and I know that Sophie's right, but it doesn't assuage my own guilt. I compare my children only to their closest friends (I cannot help but think of William and Evanee as the girls' friends) and I see that they have less.

And part of me is ashamed of my human limitations. With all the grandeur, with all the devastating otherworldly completeness of my love for them, how can it be that mundane human needs cannot be conquered? Yet still I need sleep, and food, and the occasional shower. And then today I want something else, too – not a need, a want. To walk with Sophie.

There is a park, up the hill from the hospital. It spreads like a blanket across the steep flank of the hill; it is a world away from the linoleum and bleach and crumbling plaster of the Local. It has copses and fields, a kitchen garden, adventure playgrounds and curving ponds still fed by natural springs. It is a swathe of green above the hospital, above the fluorescent-lit chicken shops and bright kebab houses nearby. Next to it is a well-known cemetery, literally Dickensian, containing as it does the graves of Fanny Dickens, Charles's sister, as well as those of his parents, his wife Catherine, and his ninth child, a daughter, Dora Annie, born while he was writing *David Copperfield*. So much of the old City of London evokes Dickens as he walked, listening, studying. But here one can stand still upon his footprints, to bow one's head as he once must have, before the gravestones of those he loved. Baby Dora lived for seven months. Her birthday is 16th August, the day after William's.

We are not here for the extended Dickenses today. Sophie suggests that we visit George Eliot, and it's as good a pilgrimage as any. I've lived close by most of my life and I'd never been.

I have also never seen Sophie outside of a hospital ward. She has been to me as teachers were when I was a small child – beings who exist inside the classroom, springing into animation only when we pupils filed in. This walk is something new, an acknowledgement that our friendship is not simply one of convenience and circumstance. We are allowing each other to spill into the remaining sliver of our lives outside the NICU and, as with space, so with time. We met three and a half weeks ago, but what is now between us was forged in the frontier's white heat. In this, my new life, I have known her life-long.

It is a steep hill and we walk up it together in silence at first. It has been twenty-four days since my surgery and I am healing for I keep pace with Sophie. It feels good to move, outside, in air. A chill, insistent rain stings my face. Buses on their slow climb fill the air with diesel, and I find myself tasting the wet fumes with pleasure. A change from stifling, soporific dry heat.

We jink from the road into the park. Sophie waits until we are through the gates to share a happy, unexpected dispatch: back at the Central Hospital, Kemisha gave Evanee a bath. Together Sophie and I turn over this information. Not a medical advancement and yet, vast progress. One of

our own has leapt forward into the world of babydom –
Evanee is a step closer to splashing and bubbles, to damp
hair and warm towels and squeaking rubber ducks. Bathing
a baby is something a mother would do.

She said it was about time, Evanee's feet smelled.

Of what? I am fascinated.

Sophie takes my question as seriously as I intended it. *She
said they smelled of feet.*

We are delighted and incredulous. How clever Evanee is –
her clever little feet, behaving like feet. They have never
touched the earth, they have never worn socks or shoes, but
still. They had been in the world since July and it is now
October. Evanee has had a bath. To us, it sounds like a baptism.

Women's communion has always been seen by patriarchal
orders as suspect, dangerous; witches, threatening in their
covens. We have been taught to see one another not as allies
but as rivals: perhaps it has been to keep us from unionising.

But with us, now, we have resisted all that old, old stuff.
We have sloughed it off. There has been no rivalry among
the women of the milking shed, no cattiness. Only
sisterhood, generosity, kindness. Perhaps it was self-selecting,
among us, though it really felt as if that climate was
organically generated within the sanctuary of the room

itself, in the air of our odd mother ship, finally a sacred women's place. Occasionally there were those who did not seem attuned to its ethos, and we let them pass us by. Women are not always kind to other women (people are not always kind to other people). So it does not go without saying and therefore should be said: in the spirit of the milking shed, we are unreservedly happy for Kemisha. Her joy has brought us joy, and has fortified us. But it cannot help but give us pause to wonder, each of us. Will we ever bathe our children?

I've never thought to smell their feet.

Me neither.

Are we neglectful mothers?

Sophie considers. It is a quality I appreciate in her, that she never offers empty reflexive reassurance. Instead, a grave consideration of whatever my mad question *du jour*.

I don't think not smelling their feet constitutes neglectful mothering.

How would you even get your face near their feet? You can't stick your head through a porthole.

We ponder this for a while, and then we reach George Eliot and greet her reverentially, beneath the looming grey of her obelisk. Rare among women, she lies beneath her own words. *Of those immortal dead who live again, In minds made better by their presence.* Sophie and I have in common a devotion to Eliot, to *Middlemarch* in particular, though I have always held a slightly bashful candle for the soppier, more sentimental *Daniel Deronda*, too. To stand here stirs a vague recollection of novels, the reading of them, and the writing. But I must forget all that. For the moment too much self can only be a hindrance.

*

All day everything is wrong. The world is out of joint; it is like breathing with a chest of broken ribs. And I never realise how much it hurts until I hold one of my daughters and instantly my ribs are healed, my own lungs fill, my own pulse slows. It is meditation. She is a lesson in stillness. A flash of grace.

I remember rolling my eyes at a yoga teacher who between sequences would ask questions and then answer them herself as she paced barefoot between us, a smouldering incense stick held between her fingers like a cigarette: Where are we? *Here.* What time is it? *The time is now.* These answers seemed maddening, meaningless, deliberately challenging. Now they seem profound to me, and essential. My child is here, now, and I am with her. Where else, what else could there be? I close my eyes and the wires are gone, the cables, the sensors, the cannulas. Gone too are the incubators left and right, the IV poles and TPN machine, the screens and monitors and bustling nurses. With my eyes closed I feel only her, and the heat that moves between us. The soles of her feet side by side upon my palm.

Her arm is raised, her own palm is flat against my heart, and I want her handprint emblazoned there. She could be no one but herself; even identical twins have different fingerprints. Within this compact person she is she; the differences between my children are there to be learned, if only I may have the chance to learn them.

I have nowhere else to be. She lifts and falls with my breath, like a sailboat.

*

We have a new nurse today, Amelia. I recognise her from around the ward; she has wide-set blue eyes, a scrappy blonde ponytail dip-dyed in mint green, and a Marilyn Monroe beauty mark above her lip. She knows absolutely everything and everyone on the ward. She has, I discover, a great many strong opinions, offered without restraint.

Day Twenty-four

My goodness, Princesa, she says to B-lette. *That was not a very styleesh chat on your seester's chead, the other day. Thank goodness eet ees gone. What a cheeky bunny.*

Cheeky bunny is Amelia's version of *being naughty*, which is the neonatal intensive care nurse's term for anything ranging from 'behaving unexpectedly' to 'gravely ill'. Amelia's Buenos Aires accent is glorious, so mellifluous it sounds almost Italian. In such a voice, *not very styleesh* resounds as the ultimate condemnation.

It becomes almost immediately obvious that Amelia is exceptional, in both her practical and her holistic care. She has deft hands, meticulous standards and a keen, all-seeing eye. I discover it was she who resolved our seemingly unending vein saga with A-lette the other day; she had heard about the head cannula and come to see it for herself, and had overheard a ward round during which Deepak had surmised that it had indubitably been the right decision to insert it, but that it was unlikely to last more than a day or two. So Amelia had taken matters into her own hands. This explains why Seema, a consultant who that morning had no responsibility for us, appeared later that day, deus ex machina, to re-site the cannula.

I must tell you, the consultants here, they are all excellent.

But each one I choose for different things. For example, to Thomas I go and I say, Thomas, this bébé he looks odd to me, and everyone is saying he looks odd because he is a twenty-six weeker but I know what I know, and can you please run genetics? It is not a cheap thing to do, and no one will want to do it. But always I go to Thomas with this because I know he will listen, and he runs the tests and yes – my poor little bébé has Down's syndrome. But at least so much else makes sense, the mother can begin to understand. For cannulas I go to Seema. With her eyes closed Seema could find a vein in the leg of a fly. As she speaks she is rolling a new nest for B-lette, strong arms spinning a towel round and round. In the telling the doctors are her courtiers, poised to do Queen Amelia's bidding. I believe it. *Otherwise maybe a junior doctor comes to replace it when the scalp vein fails and we go on and on, and Anton is an excellent reg and so he could do it but Anton, he will be scared of you now, so he will not come.* I open my mouth to protest the need for this but she shrugs. *I was working that night; I saw through the glass that you were very sad. Anton will be sad he made you so sad. And so the next day I thought,* Basta. *Now it is the time for Seema.*

DAY TWENTY-SEVEN

Thursday, 29th October

'October 29, 1977. Since I've been taking care of her, the last six months in fact, she was "everything" for me, and I've completely forgotten that I'd written. I was no longer anything but desperately hers.' – Roland Barthes, *Mourning Diary*.

That's it, Roland, I think. *You totally get it.*

DAY TWENTY-EIGHT

Friday, 30th October

It has come out that today is our wedding anniversary, and Amelia doesn't like what she's seeing one bit.

Why didn't you have a lie-in this morning, she chides, nudging me. *Okay so fine, you are here now, but where are you going for dinner? It has been a month, you have earned it. Put some make-up on, have a drink, we have your princesas safe. How long have you been married?*

Today, Gabe and I have been married four years. Two were spent in Boston; Gabe completing a post doc in biostatistics while I was drinking litres of filter coffee cross-legged on the floor of our sunny South End apartment, writing my first novel. After work we would meet on the Esplanade for long walks along the Charles River or go west through the Emerald Necklace, a linked chain of Boston's green spaces, which near our apartment was little wider than a planted cycle path. Here, a nearby guerrilla knitting group, if such a thing can be said to exist, often garlanded the lampposts and bike racks with seasonally-appropriate woolly covers – candy-cane stripes at Christmas; orange and black for Halloween; red, white and blue in July. Once a bush of honeysuckle was filled with a profusion and confusion of birds: crocheted owls, flamingos, puffins.

Our local restaurant was Ethiopian and we ate large quantities of injera. In the long months of snow and ice we drank a lot of cheap Californian red in Cambridge student bars, tramping home across the Harvard Bridge in rubber-soled snow boots and ski gloves, cheeks wine-warmed and wind-burned. In summer Gabe often put our supper in a backpack and we would climb the ladder of our fire escape to lie on the unfenced slanting roof, where the cheers and whoops of Fenway Park's baseball stadium sometimes floated to us, or the faint chorus of 'Sweet Caroline', played in the eighth innings break of every game.

I cherished these long evenings. My parents too had been newlyweds in Boston and it had always been a place of mythic happiness in their narrated history, upon which we layered our own earliest stories. And then Gabe's post doc ended and we came home to London, to our oldest friends. We hoped we might have a baby. In London were the people by whose sides we planned to weather playgroups and zoo visits and Harvesters, and frigid winter swings. In London too were our sisters, poised and ready to love the child we hoped to have.

Twenty-eight days into my daughters' lives, and our families are still waiting. I picture them, a patient ring of love around our locked perimeter fence, new aunts and newly minted grandparents, together with our friends whose children hoped one day to play with ours, all of them poised to bring their blessings to these babies like the gifts of the Wise Men. Actually, I do not want to think of Wise Men, or of Christmas. It is Halloween tomorrow, though no one here has knitted jack-o'-lantern outfits for the lampposts nor indeed for the babies, which is perhaps a missed opportunity. Soon it will be November and we will still be here, days accreting, barely distinguishable but for the up-down tweaks of oxygen, or the pastry choice downstairs.

Gabe and I always swore not to lose sight of one another; that amid the raging storms of early parenthood we would cleave together, would cherish our relationship as we nurtured our new baby. But the children have swept away our former life like a tsunami. The plans we made were for that former life, with children in it. This is a new life entirely. I now suspect it would have felt that way regardless, that anyone with children would have laughed at our ignorance, our naivety. But what did we know, then?

And so we talked yesterday about our anniversary and decided that during evening handover we would just pop across the road to what may be the world's least atmospheric Japanese restaurant, probably tied with Pastry Place in the romance stakes. We didn't want to celebrate our two-ness while we are not yet quite a foursome. The mathematics of our family hurts my head, or maybe it is the geometry.

But of course Amelia is right. I am realising begrudgingly that Amelia is always right. We should go out tonight. We can eat three courses and linger over a shared dessert. If we wanted we could reel home and sleep a deep, uninterrupted sleep, and wake whenever we want (let us ignore, for the moment, the urgent pulsing heat of engorging breasts). There would be no levy for a hangover; no newborns' cry for us at home. Our childcare arrangements are flawless and will never let us down: the NHS provides round-the-clock care, they never call in sick, they never bill. They just get on with the everyday heroism of keeping our children alive, of being more competent and qualified caregivers for our offspring than we are. If anyone except a nurse had pointed this out to me I would have decked them.

Gabe comes in and begins scrubbing his hands at the isolation sink. Amelia pounces on him.

Shame on you! she cries. *Shame, shame. You are not allowed to come back after handover tonight; we will not let you in. You must take your wife out for dinner!*

I have walked away from my half-novel like a house abandoned to dereliction. But Gabe must work still, on top of all this, long hours spent hunched over his laptop in the Bedlam that is Pastry Place. I cannot imagine the psychic schism it requires. He deserves a meal out, with a wife who is at least masquerading as a normal human. We pass one another like shift workers, he arriving so that I can run down to get some lunch or express, returning so he can go back to work. There is a relentless clockwork motion to our long days and though he is often within touching distance while we hold aloft syringes of milk or change nappies side by side, still I miss him, missing the quiet space apart in which we have always been able to hold one another.

Book a table! Amelia urges, and so I smile and say, *Yes, do.*

But no funny business, yes? Amelia wags her finger at Gabe who looks up from reading a chart, for a moment genuinely bewildered. *She has just had two babies, yes?*

*

At the last minute we got into an improbably good restaurant, run by a chef famous for witty gastronomy. I have marked the occasion with an experiment: I have folded down my Marks and Spencer's High Waisted Briefs, over the waistband of my jeans. This is a surprising success; I feel positively airy and exposed around the midriff. Sex remains not only medically prohibited but entirely unthinkable. Nonetheless, I consider going so far as to apply mascara. I text Sophie: *It's our wedding anniversary. Am I the only person headed out with their high-waisted briefs folded down over the top of their jeans?*

I am also out! In the pub. Radical. Mazel tov on reaching the folding-down stage. Next stop crotchless knickers.

This message brings me untold joy. I do not need to feel guilty because Sophie is out, too! Also I am rubbing off on Welsh-born Sophie to a heart-warming, possibly alarming degree: *mazel tov* indeed.

And so here we are, Gabe and I, across a table from one another, and the soundtrack is not the locomotive ca-*thunk* of the breast pump, but low jazz trumpet and tinkling piano. On the table before us is pâté, dramatically disguised, marzipan-style, as a satsuma. The food is Talking Point food, which is a blessed relief, for all I can think to say over and over in various tones of voice is, *I can't believe we are out.* I can sense in Gabe a heroic attempt to disguise his fatigue, and I know that what he needs from me is ninety minutes of normality. This was a good idea. The nurses take care of all of us, I realise, though this should have been long ago obvious. They work tirelessly to safeguard the families into which their babies will one day be released.

I have a go at conversation. *Meat that looks like fruit!* Gabe gives me a steady look which I return with a challenging eyebrow – *what?* – until we both collapse. A month of hysteria begins to bubble forth, laughter rising within us like shaken soda. I don't even really know what is so funny but soon we are both in stitches, and Gabe is wiping tears of laughter from his cheeks, the first tears he has let fall freely. Everything is terrible and surreal and unexpected, and unexpectedly funny. I am in layered control-wear and both breasts are leaking perilously and I have forgotten how to be a person but everything will be all right, just so long as Gabe can see that I am still me, and still in here, somewhere. We each drink two confusingly savoury cocktails, very fast, and while the room spins and our ship lurches we hold hands very tightly across the expanse of white linen.

DAY TWENTY-NINE

Saturday, 31st October

Every day I come around pretending to do something useful, Deepak announced on this morning's ward round, with theatrical sorrow, *but really I am doing nothing at all; these two marvellous babies, they are doing it all. Feeding and growing, feeding and growing. Well done, darlings.*

Amelia stands proud as punch beside her charges. There's no question that these are her babies now. She has them whenever she is working, by whose arrangement I don't know.

Amelia, what are we going to do with these two ladies? Can we think about increasing their feeds?

No, says Amelia, simply. *They desaturate too much. I want to see their oxygen requirements go down some more. Not yet.*

Okay. The boss says no, so it's no. Deepak and Amelia grin at one another. *I know my place around here.*

The ward round departs. I am lying back with Celeste; Amelia is on until 8 p.m. Neither of us is going anywhere, and so we talk.

Amelia is always upbeat and professional but the truth is that she's having a difficult weekend. It is hard; her girlfriend Dawn lives in Aberdeen; they have now been in a long-distance relationship for several years. Amelia rents a single attic room in a big shared house ninety minutes from the hospital; on two nurses' salaries they cannot afford to rent their own place, and until they can live together it does not make sense for Dawn to leave her own good job as a cardiac nurse and come here. Amelia wasn't meant to be working this weekend but someone called in sick and Amelia will never let the NICU down. But her girlfriend is here, right now, alone in London, and precious hours are passing. They love each other; they miss each other; obviously when Amelia took this extra shift they had a row about it. At 9 p.m. tonight Dawn will have to be on a sleeper back to Aberdeen because she herself is working tomorrow. Amelia doesn't know when she'll be able to come back again.

Her blue eyes are swimming. *It hurts to know that she is here and I cannot see her, but what can I do? I do it for us, she knows. I want us to buy a home, so she will never have to go. She is everything. We need the money.*

I wish I could just say – *Go, go! We'll be fine! Don't worry about us, I'm sure I can figure out the oxygen canisters* – but I know she isn't here for us, exactly. Still, I will try to make her day easier by being undemanding, and when I go for lunch I resolve to bring her back a cup of sweet builders' tea, which she has trained herself to love, she says, since it is hard to find her beloved *mate cocido* in the UK. How are they to function, these soldiers, when their own lives are always being thrust into unsolicited, unwelcome perspective by the life-and-death battles of a work day? When does romance get to matter? And why are our skilled frontline caregivers paid so little that two nurses in love must live five hundred miles apart?

While Amelia measures the next feeds into syringes a message arrives from Sophie: *William is on Optiflow!!! No more CPAP hat, I can actually see his head!! He has Evan's receding hairline. Actually he looks a bit like ET.*

Me: *Hurrah! Send pics! Mine have receding hairlines too – R&W clearly a match made in heaven.*

She sends one instantly, in which William stares the camera down, slate-grey eyes filled with challenge. He has long sandy eyelashes, and one eyebrow slightly raised. He is a captivating rebel baby.

Fierce pose. He looks like a baby James Dean!

I know, she replies, *I was just saying all that other stuff to be modest. Anyway, how was wedding anniversary? Did the rolled-down pants do the trick? Are you pregnant?*

DAY THIRTY

Sunday, 1st November

Thirty days. I had hoped by now to be glamorously thin with worry, but no. Apparently worry only makes you thin if you also give up eating Minstrels.

By the way I'm fat, I text Sophie, and she writes back, *Well, I wasn't going to be the one to tell you.*

DAY THIRTY-ONE

Monday, 2nd November

Till now my children have been naked but for their nappies, and a range of hats to rival Isabella Blow. Thank goodness Gabe went in early and so was able to forewarn me – today they are both fully clothed. It is as unexpected as coming down in the morning to find the Weimaraner in a tuxedo and cravat.

Raffaella is sporting a greying white vest printed with ice-cream cones, together with a papal sort of pointed fez; Celeste is to be found curled somewhere amid the folds of a giant Babygro the colour of Pepto Bismol on whose chest,

I will discover when we rotate her, are emblazoned the words 'MUMMY'S LITTLE STAR' in Comic Sans. I presume this has all come from the painted pine chest of drawers just outside our room, a cosy piece of domestic furniture so incongruous in a waxed linoleum hospital corridor, and which contains donated prem-wear. This ranges from handmade Christmas jumpers through hand-me-downs to actual doll's clothes.

The sight of them brings an unexpected pain to my throat. It is progress: the night nurses have turned down the temperature of the incubator. But someone else had the pleasure of choosing an outfit; of swathing and swaddling my naked babes. Another hand first clothed my daughters. They will never lie naked again; getting dressed and undressed is as exhausting as anything else for them, and so our effortless hours spent skin-to-skin are probably behind us. I've grieved nothing else we've left behind. Not the jaundice lamps, the longline, the intravenous cannulas, the CPAP hat and mask – oxygen now runs to them through a fine nasal cannula, leaving visible their beautiful faces, apart from the teddy-bear stickers on each cheek that hold the wires in place. This is my first taste of regret at the passing of a stage. That is progress, too, of a sort.

In any case there's no time to have feelings, for greater developments are afoot today and I have reason to be happy: our gang is reuniting. Kemisha and Evanee are on their way from the Central Hospital to the Local. They will need this isolation room and so we are graduating, from Intensive Care to the less intensive Special Care, one floor up. Theoretically, if not geographically, we are one giant leap closer to the door.

*

It is day thirty-one and we've come up in the world. After the freight elevator of the NICU Isolation, Special Care is vast as a ballroom. It has a flood of natural light from very high windows, which creates a feeling of miniaturisation below. For the moment ours are the only babies in incubators – the other inmates lie in open cots pushed against the high walls, a massive expanse of empty floor in the middle. Victorian orphanage meets Edwardian dancehall. We are in a small glass box in the far right corner – isolation again, but this time less isolated.

Someone's eating a Danish at the nurses' desk, I message Gabe. This is radically relaxed: the NICU air of emergency has dispersed. But the biggest difference is this: here, the nurses speak of *after*. The girls need help breathing and they cannot yet feed themselves; their oxygen and NG tubes are likely to stay for a good long time. But they no longer feel in mortal threat. Raffaella weighs a hefty 1.59kgs, Celeste an equally respectable 1.53kgs. Babies in this academy are studying the arts of feeding and growing. That is their work, and it is no mean feat. But terror no longer keeps us occupied, for the terror is receding. It is permissible to believe we are one day going home.

DAY THIRTY-TWO

Tuesday, 3rd November

To mark our reclamation of Kemisha and Evanee, Kemisha, Sophie and I decide to go out for dinner. This is every bit as radical as it sounds. I got dressed with extra care this morning: only for these girls would I put on my best, most elastic leggings. We are going to the Japanese restaurant across the road, for a meal that will probably last the exact duration of the nurses' handover, and then we will go back to the hospital for vending-machine Minstrels and a nightcap cuddle. All day I felt joyful, looking forward to it. Amelia and I discussed what I should order in great detail.

She likes the miso aubergine, but also said the tuna is very good. I consult the babies. At the mention of seaweed salad Raffaella makes a wavering motion with her free arm. *Veto or endorsement?* I asked her, but she wouldn't be drawn.

I am the first to arrive. In my previous life I would have bitten my cuticles while I waited but I have not touched my nose, eyes or mouth without scrubbing my hands since my first lesson in infection control (as a result of which I have excellent nails, an unexpected, useless bonus). Sophie and Kemisha arrive together, giggling at the conclusion of an anecdote, so I sit up straighter as they unwind scarves and unpeel coats, readying myself to be fabulous company. They both look so put together and polished and a month post-partum I still feel like an unmade bed. But I don't begrudge it as I suspect them of being naturally stylish people in their real lives, and myself of resembling an unmade bed even before I had children. It is like that joke – Moishe has surgery on his elbow and asks, *Doctor, after the operation will I be able to play tennis? Of course!* the doctor cries and Moishe is overjoyed, having never known how to play tennis before.

We order two of everything, on the basis that there are three of us at the table but seven whom dinner will ultimately feed. Kemisha explains precisely how many micrograms of alcohol would be in our breast milk after a glass of wine; she instructs us not to pump until 2.5 hours after our last sip. After precisely one third of a glass of Prosecco, Sophie falls about in the most adorable giggles – we should think of some good probing questions to ask her while she is so compromised but it hardly matters, as we tell one another absolutely everything anyway. We have an excellent gossip about the nurses. It has only been twenty-four hours and Kemisha has computed a list ranked by cleanliness, attentiveness and willingness to take instruction. Sophie and I fill her in on the staff, and our paltry but fascinating insights into their lives. Deepak's household is consumed with GCSE preparation. Thomas is training for the marathon. I am worried about my sweet Amelia; long-term long distance really isn't easy. William and Evanee are both in open cots already, and my girls are not long for their incubators either, but I am anxious about the transition because our new Special Care isolation pod has its own eccentric weather system quite apart from the rest of the ward. There is a large ceiling vent through which icy Narnian winds intermittently blow. *Well, get them to fix it,* says Kemisha simply, which I genuinely hadn't considered.

We stay until our handover exile ends and a bonus half-hour beyond it. So much passes between us, above and beneath all that is said. On the way back I feel like heel-clicking and swinging round lampposts like Gene Kelly.

DAY THIRTY-THREE

Wednesday, 4th November

I am not surprised when the new mother introduces herself as Angel, for the name is tattooed, in swoops and swirls of thick black copperplate, across the knuckles of her right hand. When I popped into the parents' room she was sitting on the soft black leather sofa in a white dressing gown stamped with turquoise hearts, and a pair of fluffy snowman slippers. She has a tiny blue star tattooed on her cheekbone, like a beauty spot, and a tear slid over it. I asked her if she was okay and she said she was, she was fine, she was great, but it's just that this morning she had a baby, and today has been a bit of a headfuck.

Angel had a propulsive birth – ninety minutes from first pain to baby born, and her daughter exploded into the world on the floor of her mother's bathroom, five weeks early. The baby's fine; she is here just to be on the safe side. The hospital decided to keep Angel for the night as well, because she's so young, because she needed so many stitches, and so that the oncologists can check her over.

Last year, when she was still fifteen, Angel finished treatment for an aggressive ovarian tumour. Her pregnancy was accidental but it is a miracle, a gift from God, she says. Her mum, her nan, her brother, her boyfriend – the whole family is overjoyed about this baby. But oh, it *hurts* to sit.

My boyfriend says I can call her anything I want, she said, and her eyes brightened. *I'm going to call her something Italian.*

I told her my daughters have recently become Raffaella and Celeste and she swooned. *I want Carlotta. My mum says she'll just be Carly. But she won't.* She looked suddenly fierce and the sneer on her face, the edge to her voice made me wonder how it would be to meet Angel in other circumstances, on the bus, perhaps, or bowling down a dark street towards me with her friends. *She's my baby, and ain't no one going to call her Carly. My Carlotta.* The repetition of her daughter's name ignited something behind her eyes that I recognised, a devastating ache of love; she needed, urgently, to go to her. The sofa is very low – I offered her a hand up from its depths and she accepted, steeling herself. In mine her hand felt a girl's hand still, despite its adult adornment. *It's a really beautiful name*, I told her, pressing her inked fingers, and her face crumpled; she was too vulnerable for kindness. I put my arm around her and she began to cry against my shoulder, hard and sudden, and then in silence pulled away and shuffled out, bow-legged, left, right, left, right, a wounded cowboy with snowman feet. *Ask for more drugs*, I called after her, unable to avoid the urge to mother this child. Afterwards I worried, maybe they didn't give her pain relief for a reason; maybe that was bad advice, to a teenage cancer survivor.

Carlotta is stationed in the far corner of Special Care and late that night Angel's boyfriend comes, tall and gangling, his hair in a stubby blond ponytail, a determined wisp of moustache on his upper lip. He is pushing Angel in a wheelchair. He stands with his hands together, head bowed, like a football player listening to the national anthem, and sobs over the open cot of his bonny baby daughter. Carlotta has an apple-green dummy that she sucks vigorously, and with obvious relish. They won't be here long. I see him reach down for Angel's hand and beside their sleeping child the two teenagers are motionless, until the boy lifts his head and turns to the nurse. *Can I hold her? I need to hold her.* Carlotta is doing well. They all are. Through the glass I feel my privilege, to bear witness to the formation of a family.

DAY THIRTY-FIVE

Friday, 6th November

A girl I don't recognise is changing Carlotta's nappy in the corner and I realise, though I cannot quite fathom it, that this is Angel. I haven't seen her since the day before yesterday when her boyfriend wheeled her up. Now she is in a pair of spray-on jeans, short and deliberately frayed at the hem to show ankles as fragile as the stem of a wineglass, rising from bulky bright white trainers. When I came in this morning it was six degrees and raining sideways, but Angel is in a white cropped top, revealing an expanse of taut midriff beneath an open bomber jacket. She has the fur collar turned up around a face made older with foundation, lip gloss, Kardashian-worthy false eyelashes. Her hair is waxed back into a very high bun, a perfect kiss curl pressed to each cheek. As she bends over her daughter I can see muscles rippling across her abdomen. Amelia and I are feeding together, each holding a syringe aloft, and across the cots we look at one another in silence, a shared thought bubble hovering in the air between us. Amelia and I are the same age. Reflexively I reach to adjust the bra-height waistband of my maternity jeans.

At Angel's feet is a car seat lined with sheepskin, a fat pink plush snake wound around its handle. She's dressed up because today is a big day.

Amelia and I finish our feeds and I text Sophie: *Can we talk about the fact that Angel is wearing a white belly top? She had a baby THE DAY BEFORE YESTERDAY.*

What can I tell you? Women were meant to have babies at sixteen. Serves us right for fighting the natural order with careers etc.

She has actually and literally got a visible six pack.

It's November! She'll catch her death, tell her to put on a cardy.

I am wearing control pants, a girdle and double breast pads in my elasticated maternity bra.

Are we sexting now?

Raffaella startles awake at my snort of laughter. She gives me a dark glare – *I've got your number, lady* – then, having warned me, falls instantly and completely back to sleep. Outside, Angel and Carlotta and the boyfriend are leaving. Through my glass pod I blow them a kiss, but Angel doesn't once look back.

DAY THIRTY-SIX

Saturday, 7th November

Today the stainless-steel trolley on which the notes are kept is immediately outside the door of isolation, so I flick through Celeste's observations before washing my hands a second time, to enter our pod and see the girls.

Self-ventilating in ass, it says, and so little surprises me any more that for a moment I think, *Well, why not?* Then I realise that the night nurse's handwriting leaves something to be desired. In air. My daughter is breathing alone, in air. I send a rapturous dispatch to Gabe and his reply confirms my own suspicions.

It has been clear for some time that she is a genius.

DAY THIRTY-SEVEN

Sunday, 8th November

The girls are thirty-six weeks plus two days, today. They weigh 1.73kg and 1.67kg, respectively. Today is Day Thirty-seven. Marking one or all of these occasions, someone has given us cardigans. All around the ward parents are arriving to discover them like Christmas presents, tiny, exquisite, handmade garments for no reason other than random kindness. I hope our pleasure in them is reported back to our invisible benefactors. Small acts of random kindness happen over and over here: life-affirming; soul-enriching. Thank you, strangers. Whenever we have fallen, hands have caught us.

Raffaella's is white, in a pattern of elm leaves and eyelets. It has many tiny buttons gleaming down the middle, like oyster shells. It is Victorian in its high neckline, its elaborate prim laciness. Celeste has a heartier number, a chunkier cable knit, in a wheaty, oatmealy colour. Raffaella's is for a Victorian child to sit for a cameo; Celeste's is for toasting marshmallows before a Scandinavian log fire. I decide to put them on immediately. The traditional enlivening arctic air blasts from the vent above us, and so each is already in a long-sleeved vest, a long-sleeved Babygro and a knitted hat, and lies tucked to the chin beneath several layers of folded monkey-printed muslin and a final layer of blanket (also hand knitted, also a gift).

In their cardigans they are so padded with insulating layers that their arms stick directly out at an unyielding ninety degrees. They look like scarecrows, or like cruciform papoose babies, or maybe the *Angel of the North*, but in any case they are still asleep, and it was a job to get them on, so I am not taking them off again.

DAY THIRTY-EIGHT

Monday, 9th November

My poor Amelia. Long-distance is too hard, too unpredictable, too expensive. Their lives will pass while they wait for one another; two Penelopes. Dawn is home in Aberdeen, and isn't coming back.

It's a bright day; cold winter light floods our little box as we change nappies, side by side. *I love her*, Amelia says simply. Her wide blue eyes fill. *I don't know how to be, now.*

There is nothing to say. They sounded right for each other, these two. The most prosaic obstacles have felled a true romance – money, geography, time.

What will you do?

I will work, she says, *and she will work. And we will both be very sad.* She bends over, giving her full attention to the miniature vest she's popping up, one, two, three. Then she pats the baby on the tummy, strokes her downy head. *But look at you, my cheeky Celeste, you are self-ventilating. So life is not so very bad.*

My first thought is to text my sisters-in-law to demand a Rolodex of glamorous and eligible London-based women. I would love to be the one to return our wise, generous Amelia to happiness, to care for her as all day she cares for others. But immediately I think, that wouldn't be the way. It feels wrong even to have considered another woman when Amelia's true love is just there, a few hundred miles north, irretrievable.

DAY THIRTY-NINE

Tuesday, 10th November

Something about Dawn and Amelia's separation feels deeply wrong to me. I text Sophie, *I'm pretty sure that it would all be fine if everyone just gave up their petty attachment to free will and allowed me to be in charge of absolutely everything.* I think for a minute and then, as if she might have power to authorise this new regime, add the clarification, *Except my own life, that's too hard. You have to make all my decisions while I'm sorting out everyone else.*

You've got the wrong girl, she answers, *I can't even decide which tights to wear today. I don't remember how to do this.*

What sort of tights would a normally functioning human woman wear?

Sophie has a job interview today, for an internal change of position.

Black, it's mid-November. And wear comfortable shoes, so you're not distracted. You'll wow them, I know it. Coffee?

Yes but do not let me have a cursed pastry or I will vomit on the interviewer.

At least they would remember you.

Actually, let's do afterwards – I need to prep.

See you on the other side. You are smart and brave and competent and insightful and committed, they'd be mad not to snap you up. I bet you're brilliant at … whatever it is that senior charity executives do.

I am indeed quite brilliant at all the things that senior charity executives do. Whether I am currently capable of communicating that fact, or indeed any fact, remains to be seen. You may buy me a free coffee when I return, if you like.

In my current suspension of recognisable reality, I experience it as an unwelcome intrusion when forced to make small talk with the girl at Pastry Place. I cannot imagine the full-beam spotlit assault of a job interview. Parents whose children lie in hospital limbo should not have to go to job interviews. We should not have to go to supermarkets or offices or on public transport or anywhere at all without the buffer of an explanation. *Cheer up, love*, advises bus driver after bus driver. A lapel pin would do as well: *NICU Day 39*.

It is everyone else's ward round on Special Care, and to pass my exile I am mixing a Nescafé in the parents' kitchen. Today someone has donated some mini bags of salted Hula Hoops: we are easily pleased here, so this is tantamount to a festival. As I eat breakfast Hula Hoops from my fingertips, I compose a letter of recommendation to Sophie's potential future boss. I am, after all, a current colleague.

Over the 39 days that I have known her, Sophie Parr has shown exceptional fortitude and a soldier's courage. She is a startlingly quick learner, manages resources efficiently, and is excellent at time management under even the most unpromising circumstances. In her own 84 days of NICU service thus far she has completed Ph.D.-level literature reviews of various subjects including but not limited to: Gavage Feeding the Ventilated Infant; Kangaroo Care: Its Practical Application within a High-Tech NICU Environment; CPAP or Optiflow: Make Your Bloody Mind Up, Guys. She is also a master at orienteering, having timed, to the nearest half-minute, the quickest walk between her empty flat and the bedside of her hospitalised son. She is a powerful lobbyist. She is a tireless worker. Her hobbies include pumping breast milk; opening chocolate Penguins one-handed while pumping breast milk; telling startlingly filthy jokes at odds with her conker-haired, doe-eyed appearance, all while pumping breast milk. Also she turns up, and turns up, and she keeps turning up. It should be noted that this is hard: not everyone keeps turning up, and we do not judge those who can't, because they can't. Sophie Parr turns up.

I hope that interviewer knows the calibre of human being that she has in her office.

*

Later a message comes through from Kemisha. *S. back and she looks in pieces. Pastry Place in ten?*

We don't order anything, but we sit down at a rickety bar-height table. We imagine we know, and we are waiting for Sophie to speak.

I got the job, she says softly, and then she buries her head in her hands and sobs, a naked despair I have never yet seen in her, and Kemisha and I put a hand on each of her shoulders and find we have taken one another's hands, too, across the table; a ring of silent support around one of our own. We have a woman down; like American footballers, we will stay motionless until our teammate rises.

We can all say it now, the three of us, Sophie, Kemisha and me – we don't yet know when, but our four children, sooner or later, will come home. What a thing. And now Sophie has raised a periscope and has seen what lies ahead, over the next horizon. New understanding that soon will touch us all.

Our children will be discharged and this suspension of reality will end, and with the inrush of daily life and daily motherhood we will have our babies with us and still, sometimes, we will have to be apart from them. We three have jobs, and must work. We three have lives, and we must remember how to live them.

One day Sophie will bring William home and there she will hold him close, to try to heal the wound of this long separation. But months of her maternity leave have slipped by in this place, and are passing still. After fighting so long, the thought of ever again leaving him in someone else's care is intolerable. Better to have flunked the interview. Better to fear unemployment and penury, just for the moment, to stave off imagining future separations.

DAY FORTY

Wednesday, 11th November

In a bleak photograph towards the end of *Hold Your Prem* by Jill Bergman, a mother is captured 'At Home', a term that puts me in mind of one of Anna Pavlovna's salons each time I read it. Debrett's notes that when one hosts a luncheon or supper party, one's guests should receive cards 'engraved in script from a copperplate', going on to provide the clarifying information that 'the "a" for "at" is in fact lowercase, and only the "H" for "home" is uppercase'. Our infelicitous capitalisation makes all the difference.

The *salonnière* in Jill Bergman's photograph has no guests, but has acquired for herself a supportive nursing chair much like those on the ward, the only evidence of her baby a white woolly hat beneath the mound of her unflattering shirt. It seems the major development from 'In Hospital' to 'At Home' is the dinner plate balanced inconveniently upon the woman's thighs, just beyond the heap of infant. Her legs are up on a footstool like those of a recovering invalid, her shoes projecting unhygienically close to the knife and fork held by a man who sits cross-legged at her feet who has – inexplicably – no plate or food of his own. This, then, is the happy homecoming: a life spent sweating semi-recumbent against synthetic leather, a future of makeshift TV-style dinners that your chairless partner must watch you eat, from below. But what is At Home to us? We have now been in hospital forty days.

I refuse to come over all biblical and make anything of it, and instead I shall use this landmark to look on the bright side. Stockholm syndrome: count me in! I shall love my captors, and sing their praises.

I am bored out of my skull, it's true, but I have been led to believe that that is par for the course, with new motherhood. Life with newborns is meant to be intellectually arid and exhausting and tedious and repetitive, so in that sense my first forty days have conformed entirely to expectation. Presumably I would also have been intermittently terrified, and overwhelmed, too. But I have sought out an upside to our incarceration.

With the end of the cohabiting extended family, most British women now bring babies home to solitude, very quickly left by their working menfolk to go quietly mad. Each is cut off from her peers, further isolated by the toxic myth that these early weeks should be a blissful time of unambivalent sensual bonding, complete emotional fulfilment, and the casual barefoot baking of sourdough or brownies in one's copious spare time. Instead, they are mostly left with only their squalling babies for company, trailing in desperate dressing gowns through a tide of discarded muslins and Dairy Milk wrappers. In suburbs and in high-rises, women at their most vulnerable are alone.

While I express I read Adrienne Rich, furiously highlighting line after line: *The worker can unionise, go out on strike; mothers are divided from each other in homes, tied to their children by compassionate bonds; our wildcat strikes have most often taken the form of physical or mental breakdown. For mothers, the privatisation of the home has meant not only an increase in powerlessness, but a desperate loneliness …*

Well. Nothing about my new parenthood is privatised (or for that matter private). Powerless, maybe, but there is no desperate loneliness At Home for me. I get dressed every single morning. I have colleagues! I have office gossip. I have an actual and literal water cooler at which to exchange it. For the first time in my life I no longer suffer the secret fear that everyone else is together at Central Perk, without me. The Neonatal Intensive Care Unit is Central Perk and here I am, on the orange velvet sofa, with Sophie on one side, Kemisha on the other. New mothers need support and sorority, companionship and wise women, and here I have all these, in spades.

Whatever. In Hospital is clearly the superior way to do it.

DAY FORTY-ONE

Thursday, 12th November

Today it is my six-week check-up. For a brief period this afternoon, I am once again to be the patient. I had thought that the extended hospitalisation of my two infants would immunise me against prurient speculation but no, today all the nurses are nudge-nudge, wink-winking. No fewer than three staff members have independently told me the same cautionary tale: the young couple they had here who fell pregnant, accidentally, before their first premature baby was discharged; siblings, gestationally, only seven months apart. *And then,* says Amelia darkly – and even on what was now the third telling of this story I was again floored by the punchline – *it was triplets, and we had them all back here. They now have four in the same school year. You will ask the doctor for a coil, yes?*

My check-up is unremarkable. My scar is healing well; my abdominal muscles have separated but hopefully over time will find their way back to one another, weary old friends. I am released to drive, and to begin light exercise. The obstetrician cannot explain why I began to haemorrhage at twenty-nine weeks. Maybe multiple pregnancy. Maybe advanced maternal age. Maybe … maybe some misalignment of the stars. If I were to get pregnant, I am given a one-in-ten chance that something similar would happen again.

In these last weeks I have felt an intense longing to be pregnant again. I want it some days more than can possibly be rational – the urge is so strong that it sets off alarm bells in an executive, monitoring level of my brain that takes the temperature of my mind and then advises, *Hold on a sec here, something is a bit out of whack.* Perhaps it is hormones – some muddled cocktail of an interrupted gestation, and post-partum oxytocin thwarted by the nightly routine trauma of separation. Perhaps it is an urgent psychological need for a corrective experience. Next time I would be sensible, I tell myself. I would conceive only one child at a time; I would not be so amateurish as to haemorrhage. I would give birth at forty weeks to a big baby who would breathe deep lungfuls of new air without struggle, slick with her own newness, skin to skin against my chest.

I think these things in earnest – as if I could, by dint of will, make them happen. One gets a second chance so rarely in life; I would not let this one slip through my fingers. But of course it wouldn't be a second chance. Another pregnancy cannot return to my daughters our lost months of togetherness. It is they to whom I wish to give this restoration, to whom I want to give that strength to gasp their own first heady breath. I want to start again and give them everything I am and have, a coiled unity restored to us so that I might once again pulse my own lifeblood into them but next time do it better; blood and oxygen and iron and strength and dizzying breathless love. They, and not some third stranger-baby. But the urge to feel my belly taut with child again does not diminish, even when this penny drops.

I just want to be able to mother my children, I text Sophie.

She writes back, *I just want to hold my son, and watch Bake Off.*

That's it, I think. I have not yet held a baby at the same time as a digestive biscuit and a cup of tea.

DAY FORTY-TWO

Friday, 13th November

I have become institutionalised, I know, but mostly I have
no wish to fight against it because it numbs my hardest
feelings and thereby helps me function. My daughters need
me sane and steady. And we are expected by the staff to
remain jolly and indefatigable – there is no clear sense, here,
that to grieve would in fact be normal, human, rational. Too
much sadness would draw the psychs and the social workers
('In their long coats, Running over the fields'), wondering
whether I was perhaps, *not up to it* or maybe just *not
managing*. I must not ululate, or rend my hair. Therefore I

cannot think too freely about the deprivation that is my children's earliest babydom. I must not tally the hours they lie untended, nor permit myself to imagine their new neurological systems busily organising and extrapolating from the lessons of Intensive Care into an understanding of the world beyond it. Nearing footsteps and a hand extended often means a blood test: touch is very often restraint, and pain. They should still be *in utero* but already suffering and loneliness are their old friends, and so is fear. Crying does not always summon comfort – I don't know if the nurses go to them when they are frightened, late at night. Sorrow is not a medical need. I cannot change these things, am not permitted to call them the barbarisms that they are, and so as not to be labelled mad for pointing at the horror of it all, for fracturing what is surely pluralistic ignorance, I don't allow myself to see. But every now and again something will jar me, and today it was the fingernails.

At birth they had none. Now – a triumph! – their fingernails have reached the end of their fingertips, an index of our time here, which at present is forty-two days. Raffaella's rice-grain thumbnail is quite sharp and she has a hair-fine line across one cheek where she has scratched herself, red and rising now into a hive. I mentioned it to

Noor who said, looking embarrassed, that we aren't allowed to bring in baby clippers. *Some mums file them.* She could see that something about this suggestion had upset me and offered an alternative. *Some people find it easier just to bite them down.*

The word *allowed* struck me like a pebble. What kind of mothers are not *allowed* to cut their children's nails? Dangerous mothers who can't be trusted. Mothers must not be left to care for tiny toes and fingers. All the health and safety regulations of the ward, all the rational justifications for this edict cannot alter the fact that I am a mother whose access to and interaction with her children is meted out by the absolute authority of a hospital: theirs to give and theirs to take away. A chance change in policy controls the manner in which I am allowed to touch, feed, hold and speak to my own daughters. What little I have of them is only because it is permitted.

I choose the intimacy and expediency of my teeth over the Sisyphean and humiliating task of filing forty microscopic nails. Still. No sharp objects. I may love and respect my warders, but there's no denying that we are in prison.

DAY FORTY-THREE

Saturday, 14th November

It is Evanee's due date today. She has reached the grand old age of forty gestational weeks. For Kemisha, today should have been long walks, hot curries and chunks of pineapple – a recipe for heartburn in the heavily pregnant woman if ever I have heard one. Kemisha should be gearing up to meet her daughter but instead they are already old friends; Evanee was born sixteen weeks ago, in high summer. Now it is mid November. All over the city, the Christmas lights are up.

Sophie and I have talked a lot about the ambivalence of our impending due dates. Gratitude that our children have survived to such a landmark will mingle with a grief that feels inevitable. For us it cannot but be a trigger for all the ways in which our pregnancies diverged from expectation; a time to consider the manner in which our children's lives resemble all we'd hoped for them, or don't.

And then there is Kemisha. She is – I feel quite confident saying this – capable of a happiness I cannot imagine. She has approached the day with characteristic and – to me, startling – optimism. She is robust, and defiant. Defiant is the word that I see most clearly when I think of her. Today, she has decided, is Evanee's due date but also – as should have been technically the case – her birthday; and a birthday should be celebrated in style. Kemisha has brought in a tiny dress for the girl of the hour, a flounced navy blue confection with white polka dots and matching bloomers, and she herself is dressed up for a party. She has a gift for her daughter, and a cake, which is beautiful. It is big enough to share amongst her family and friends who come in a steady, interchanging stream all day, somehow, despite the winter visiting restrictions. In lilac and yolk-yellow, HAPPY DUE DATE, EVANEE. She has brought in her proper SLR camera and in the many photos it will be almost impossible to believe this celebration was in the isolation ward of an intensive care unit. Kemisha has made of her due date a beautiful landmark. This is the true birthday gift.

I had always assumed my own due date would be a day on which I couldn't help but think of how things *should* have been. But watching Kemisha I think, What is *should*? There is no other world but this one; hers is the fuller acceptance of reality, and within it a celebration that her daughter has survived to see a date that looked, when she came into the world in July, to be impossible. Is it because she is so young? I really don't think so, for there is not a streak of naivety in her. She is wise and brave and fearless. She just – *chooses*.

DAY FORTY-FOUR

Sunday, 15th November

Gabe has struck up a friendship with a father on the ward, which means they know neither each other's name nor the names, genders or conditions of each other's incarcerated children, but that they now exchange three sentences while hand washing, instead of the more traditional one. To Sophie and Kemisha I have exposed myself while I have exposed myself; over the whirr and click and drip of breast pumps we have cried and cackled, confessed and commiserated. But for Gabe, after forty-four days, this man offers a new experience of intimacy and connection here.

This nameless father has had a baby in Neonatal Intensive Care before, and is therefore both realistic and inspiring. He is Kenny Rogers' Gambler on the train, dispensing wisdom, promising an ace that we can keep. Today, while he and Gabe soaped, they discussed boxing.

The talk is of an upcoming fight between the UK's Tyson Fury and Ukrainian Wladimir Klitschko, the long-reigning World Heavyweight Champion. Born into a family of Gypsy bare-knuckle fighters, Fury was, this veteran father told Gabe, born three months early, and was not expected to live. He weighed a single pound.

Later, I would discover that I found almost everything about Tyson Fury to be repellent and reprehensible, from his veneration of his own namesake, Mike Tyson, to his flamboyant homophobia, his unabashed sexism, his uniformly antediluvian posturing. But none of this diminishes the fact that one dark weekend that November, when the wards were all shutting up against influenza and a plague of chicken pox was rumoured to be ravaging the borough, I sat in Special Care and on my phone I studied photographs of his body, learning his shape, his lines, like a proud new lover. He was a gift, from Gabe's nameless friend to Gabe, from Gabe to me, and I handed him onwards to

Sophie and Kemisha, with love. We marvelled over the mountainous biceps, the triumphant sheen of sweat, the conqueror's grin. His thick wrists are free of cannulas. His flared nostrils are self-ventilating, in air. In the photo, Fury stands at six foot nine, and weighs 117 kilos, all of it pure, solid hope. What else weighs 117 kilos, I wondered? A car? An ox? A mountain?

DAY FORTY-SIX

Tuesday, 17th November

It is party season, it seems. Today is World Prematurity Day, a red ring on the calendar that for the previous thirty-five years has passed me by. To mark the occasion the hospital charity will host a tea party in the hallway of Special Care, attended by former inmates and their parents. There has been mounting excitement among the staff. This, after all, is a rare glimpse at the bigger picture, and a sweet reward – a triumphant parade of two- and five- and eight- and twelve-year-olds whose lives they have saved, in past years. When I arrived this morning Chantal and Pam were up on office

214

swivel chairs in the hallway, sticking up bunches of royal blue and purple balloons with surgical tape. Pam has got a Prematurity Awareness pin beside the nurse's watch on her chest. Chantal's hair is in short schoolgirl bunches, each tied with a wide purple ribbon, in a long, floppy bow. There is a festive air.

I'm dying to see Baby Yang, Chantal calls, and Pam squeals, *Ooh, do you think they'll come?*

Mum said she would. And Noor told me that Hansel and Gretel are definitely on the list.

Usually my curiosity can be piqued by human-interest stories – Hansel and Gretel: ward nicknames or actual names? They've had three pairs of Ronnie and Reggie's, so anything's possible – but today I don't care. In my ears these names resound and I hear only, *germs, germs, germs. Influenza. Chicken pox. RSV. Plague.* I am in a poisonous mood, and have lost the vestiges of the sense of humour I have grappled back, week by week. What are they all thinking? Has it all, till now, just been an elaborate role-playing exercise? Are we not, then, mortally worried about RSV? Why the endless disinfecting, why the visiting ban, why the hygiene protocols and isolation elevator and outdoor clothes to be left by the door if once a year it is all suspended? *Throw caution to the wind, never mind all that, today!* The ward has been in winter lockdown, and all of a sudden it will be swarming with giant children smearing icing and cake crumbs and a smorgasbord of deadly cold viruses on to every surface of the hallway. Have I been washing my flayed hands to bleeding just for kicks? This afternoon tea is an affront to every axiom. Something about it has tipped me over the edge.

It is possible, I concede, that my rage has been stoked by something else. Envy is the most likely candidate. Envy and the fear that we will never leave, that I will never get to button two excitable little moppets into party frocks and bring them back here for a victory tour of the rooms where once they lived. Instead, I will be forced to elbow my way through this fiesta every November for the rest of my life: *Excuse me, excuse me, I must get to the isolation room at the back, my daughters are turning thirty.*

I storm through the main ward of Special Care to discover that Raffaella and Celeste have each given us a box of Milk Tray wrapped in shiny purple paper, the colour of Prematurity Awareness (who knew?). The chocolates are arranged at the foot of each cot, with cards addressed to Mummy and Daddy. The long-ago adverts rise effortless and unbidden: the handsome daredevil scaling buildings, and all because the lady loves Milk Tray. I cannot help myself. For a moment I picture the girls scaling the outside of their Perspex hospital cots, tiny abseilers risking life and limb to give us these tokens. No child should ever have to thank their parents for giving birth to them; Winnicott is very clear on this point. Children, after all, do not ask to be born. My bad mood has loosened my self-control, has compromised my defences and made me vulnerable to sentiment. As a result, these ridiculous cutesy cards – *Love from Raffaella*; *Love from Celeste* – have undone me. It is 8 a.m. and I am weeping as I hold syringes of milk aloft above my sleeping daughters while with the other hand I am stuffing Surprise Parcels and Caramel Charms into my mouth, one after another, barely pausing to chew. You are not, obviously, allowed to eat on the ward. But why would it matter? Everyone else is breaking the rules today.

*

I have had to get a grip, because the nurses are in a state of such innocent excitement that I owe them at the very least the concealment of my hostility, if not a veneer of actual enthusiasm. I keep studying them for signs of irony or artifice but have found none. *Are you coming to the party?* someone will ask, if you so much as step out to go to the loo. *Don't forget the party!* they will call, if you duck into the kitchen to microwave a pot of baked beans.

In the lobby of the ward there are twenty, maybe twenty-five adult people. I raise my chin in defiance; I refuse to look at or acknowledge the existence of the pint-sized ones. A purple-clad trestle table stands in front of the parents' lounge on which stand cartons of orange juice, a tub of cherry tomatoes, a plate of Dairy Lea sandwiches, three tubes of salt & vinegar Pringles and several open bowls of crisps. Someone in a purple charity T-shirt holds aloft a box of cheese straws and announces that they are just over here, if anyone needs one for a toddler. Do toddlers have a thing for cheese straws? *Well,* I think bitterly, hamming it up for my own benefit, *I wouldn't effing know, would I?* On a teetering cardboard stand are cupcakes topped with swirls of lilac buttercream and glitter and crested with a pair of fondant baby feet, as if a very tiny baby was submerged, head-first, in the icing. At the centre of all this excess is a large rectangular cake on which is surreally printed 'HAPPY WORLD PREMATURITY DAY, 17th NOVEMBER'. It is very white and very large and elaborately frosted and scalloped, like a wedding cake.

Much later the filthy hordes have departed and the nurses and volunteers are sweeping up the debris. I have boycotted both the setting-up and the dismantling. On principle I have helped not at all. I am safe here in my glass box at the back, and nothing would induce me to go back out there until the bunting and streamers and posters are packed away. In the doorway Noor appears and gives me a long look. Then she disappears and returns with a cupcake. *I ate the baby feet off it for you*, she says, matter- of-factly. *Take it home. They're good, my sister-in-law made them.* She is gone before I can thank her but I wrap the cupcake in paper hand towels and stuff it into my bag, next to the one I had already hate-swiped, earlier.

*

I can't remember the last time I had to set an alarm. Every night between 2 and 3 a.m. my body rouses me and I am sitting up in bed, pulling my tangled hair back from my face before I realise I'm no longer dreaming. Beside me Gabe is motionless in deep sleep. When the noise of the breast pump begins he will stir and turn, but for now the only sound is of his breath.

There is a presumed hierarchy of suffering in our world; fathers expected to keep working, to keep smiling, to 'support' their wives or girlfriends, though the children in peril are theirs just as they are ours. Such is the language. Gabe goes to the hospital early mornings, returning every afternoon, and each daytime visit the nurses will coo, *Gosh, what a good Daddy you have, lucky girls*, though I am there with them from dawn to nightfall, un-cooed. The men win praise for very little, but the cost of this low bar is high. They must be fine, fine, fine. They must be squiring robots, and peripheral. Even if he didn't have to work, even if we were able to keep exactly the same hospital hours, it would be assumed by almost everyone both inside and outside of the hospital that Gabe suffered less than I.

I can do all this by feel, now, but I put on my glasses so I can see Gabe's face. He is in there, somewhere, dreaming. He has barely cried through these months. How is he, really? Does he believe that the best way of caring for me is to shield me from his own fear, his own anxiety? And if so, where does he take it? Where can it go? A few nights ago he shouted in his sleep, a sudden, incoherent roar of fury, and then lapsed into silence though his fists were clenched, a man at war. In the morning I asked if he had had a nightmare but he said he didn't remember, he didn't think so, and would I like him to bring up a cup of tea?

By the sodium orange wash of the streetlight that falls through the gap in the curtains, and by the tiny green LED on the front of the pump, I assemble, connect, switch on. Tuck duvet high up, between bottles and belly. Start the timer. Switch on the pump – click, click, thunk. Phone the ward. The usual routine. Beside me Gabe buries his face in the pillow for a moment, turns, and lays a sleep-heavy hand on my thigh. I resist the urge to whisper a hello, for if I talk to him he wakes up to reply. If I am silent he will be asleep again in moments. One thing I do know, he is very tired.

Tonight it is Jamila who answers. She was so happy to be assigned to the girls, she tells me – she hasn't had them in weeks and they are almost unrecognisable. It must be calm and quiet on the unit, because she is ready to chat. *They're proper babies now*, she tells me, pride in her voice. *They're so big! I couldn't believe it when I weighed them. 2.032kgs and 1.852kgs.* She laughs. My head throbs as it always does, a rich, midnight ache. Reports of them make me feel as if they are receding from me. Still, I will never forget that it was Jamila who first helped me nurse my babies. On other nights, I have lain awake in misery after this call – the night nurse a brusque stranger from an agency, or one of very few people on the ward with whom I do not feel a connection, whose handling irritates or jars me. I am grateful when it is Jamila.

How are they?

There is a long pause.

They're right as rain in themselves, she says finally. *You're not to worry. I couldn't believe it when I saw the pair of them, both self-ventilating, and their sats have been perfect all night, they've done so well, clever girls. But tonight they've not had the easiest time, to be honest. They're sleeping now, but we've had a lot of tears. They miss their mummy. Miss Celeste in particular has been telling us all about it. Well, they've got a point. They're doing so well now, and mostly they just need you, really, don't they?*

I whisper my thanks and drop the phone into my lap. Tha-*thunk*, tha-*thunk*. Tha-*thunk*, tha-*thunk*.

They're doing so well.

They just need you, really, don't they?

Tomorrow will be the forty-eighth day that I have been separated from my children. For forty-nine days a part of my mind has absented itself, a necessary auto-lobotomy, grief neatly excised in order that I might survive the quotidian inhumanity of separation. To leave each night I must crush an ever-rising instinct. *It's where they need to be; you need your strength; you cannot sleep on the waxed linoleum floor nor will they let you.* Now I find that these facts have been emptied of meaning. Day by day I have been learning to be a mother, but what a twisted, will-o'-the-wisp mother I now see reflected: some horror from a German fairy tale. When night falls I am something else entirely: a yearning spirit with empty arms.

And Raffaella and Celeste? How are those two forming souls to comprehend what it is to have a mother? By day she is all song and tenderness; she is milk and promise. But then night creeps in and with the light she leaves, and though we cry for her she never comes. The promises are empty.

Everything is wrong.

They're doing so well.

Everything is broken.

They just need you, really, don't they?

Something within me snaps. I feel it, like a ligament. Like a heartstring.

DAY FORTY-SEVEN

Wednesday, 18th November

This morning I am possessed. I have in mind that it is Lilith: she-demon, thief of newborn babies; proto-feminist; one of the world's most ancient female spirits newly rehabilitated as an icon among contemporary scholars of Jewish egalitarianism. In some tellings, Lilith was Adam's first wife, made from earth as he was, and therefore unwilling to accept submission. Cursed by angels, pregnant women have feared her as a baby-snatcher but my heart is in accord with her sisterly reclamation, in admiration of her courage, her rebellion, her voice. She has come to represent a stand against systematic patriarchal repression, and she has a dark sensuality that seems in truer accord with the dark sensuality and power of motherhood. I feel her burning behind my own eyes, and welcome her. I call upon the patron saint of baby-snatchers. There can be no return, now, from this place of righteous anger.

*

It is Thomas on ward round, and my resolve falters. He has not been our consultant since the night he saw me weeping over the golden glitter-dust of Raffaella's shaved hair (which has, incidentally, not grown back in the last month, though the spider-silk blonde hair on the other side is longer. Half of her head still gleams, hairless as a polished apple). Since then I have been awkward with him when we've met in passing, over-keen to show myself as rational, as Not Depressed, and, initially, to disguise the fact that I was fantasising about running a cannula into his head, ungently. During these exchanges I have heard myself vacuous and twittery – murderous disguised with unthreatening girlishness. It is fair to say that Thomas has not seen me at my best. I'm fairly sure he thinks I am a maniac or an emotional wreck, or both.

Thomas has quite the entourage, today. There are two senior registrars: Anton, who has a new pair of rather dashing Harry Potter tortoiseshell glasses, and a tall, saturnine woman with a yellow and red owl-shaped handbag. What do the female consultants keep in their handbags, I always wonder? And if it is essential, then how do the male consultants do without? Behind them there are two junior doctors, and a young Nigerian medical student who glanced in alarm at the warnings of our contagion plastered on our isolation door and now stands rigid with the folded-in posture one might adopt in the Harrods china department. *Come, come, nothing to be scared of here*, I want to reassure her. *What's a touch of ceftazidime-resistant pseudomonas between friends?* Noor is there, as she is our nurse today. And Thomas – rather oddly – also seems to have a very small nun in tow.

It is to the nun that I am first introduced, Sister Eucharia, who is visiting the unit from Uganda. Thomas is courtly with her, which I find begrudgingly endearing. *It is a true blessing to have twins*, she tells me, and I nod. *Yes*, I say, *hello, Sister*, and I am opening my mouth to ask a polite question about her work in Uganda when the thought drops into my mind, round and distinct as a penny – *I don't care*. I am unable to keep up the pretence of social niceties when they stand between me and my single, fixed objective. Over Sister Eucharia's head, I fix my gaze upon Thomas, expecting objection, or resistance. 'I am taking these babies home. With feeding tubes. It's enough.'

The close air thickens. I spoke too loudly and our tiny elevator is taut, suddenly, with tension. Eight people are staring at me. I am known on the ward. Amenable, agreeable, self-effacing. It is as if a houseplant had begun to assert itself. There have been signs, subtle and moon-slow, of change within me. Increasingly I raise a tentative finger and say *hello*, and *excuse me*, and *perhaps we might consider* … But now, today, I am at war with everybody and it is in my voice, my eyes. All these good kind people. With infinite care and patience have they grown my almost-children into babies, have they fed and washed them, ministered and medicated and given breath to their lungs and been, by virtue of their incomparable and essential expertise, a constraint upon my own burgeoning state of motherhood. I have done with them.

Thomas turns to Noor, and when I glance at her I see her leaning in the doorway, arms crossed, eyebrows raised to him in challenge. A slow smile is forming. Thomas turns back to me.

'Okay,' he says, and I see stars.

In the doorway Thomas turns. 'I'll examine them tomorrow; let's not wake them now. I'll talk to the discharge team. It takes a few days because you'll have to room in, so let's get this rolling.'

It takes time for the crowd to disperse as, having washed their way in, they must each wash their hands again to exit. Last to leave, Sister Eucharia is still smiling and shaking her head in agreement with something – with me, with Thomas, with the rightness of a transformation that, however inelegantly, has finally taken place. She has sensed it. No one usually touches me in here, in my isolation room – ceftazidime-resistant pseudomonas is the best of what patients in this pod usually carry. But when they leave she squeezes my hand.

Both girls have slept through their mother's big moment, so they will have to take my word for it. I check the charts. I line up syringes of medication. Raffaella doesn't stir as I attach a syringe to her NG tube and aspirate just enough to daub a drop on to pH paper and check its acidity, and then I attach her second or perhaps her third breakfast. I remove the plunger with a practised thumb and hold the milk low over her cot. There is silence, only the soft smooching sound of Celeste sucking contentedly on her miniature dummy.

This is it, girls, I tell them. *You're being baby-snatched. We can do this. Look at us – we're doing it.*

DAY FORTY-EIGHT

Thursday, 19th November

On this morning's ward round Thomas examined them and paused for a long time with his stethoscope. Jolly chat about our homecoming was suspended while he ordered scans for this afternoon. Echocardiograms took place within hours, revealing that both twins have holes in their hearts. I am standing absolutely still between their cots, one hand resting lightly on each chest as it rises and falls. Thomas is coming back to talk to me.

It occurs to me, almost as if in passing, that I am very tired. I want someone to explain to me what just happened.

I want to hand over the last half-hour to Sophie or to Kemisha for them to parse it using their own instincts, and then feed back to me what to do and how to feel, an external, outsourced part of my own nervous system. Emotional dialysis.

Thomas found holes in their hearts.

Kemisha replies instantly. *ASD? VSD? PFO?*

A moment later Sophie adds, *Pastry Place?*

I couldn't leave until I'd seen Thomas but when he came he was full of reassurance. He is perfectly happy with the echocardiograms: we have the good kind of murmur, apparently. A large minority of healthy adults are walking around with just such heart-holes; extended hospitalisation and repeated examination means we learn more about the inner workings of these babies than by rights we ought; we uncover secrets that should not be our business. More information is not necessarily better. I am meant – and he advises this in all seriousness – to forget all about it, and get on with the rare and precious business of being happy, and preparing to go home. I didn't really follow his explanation or acronyms, but I know Kemisha will explain it to me later.

Over coffee, Dr Kemisha reiterates Thomas's assertion that I don't need to worry. So once I have recovered from the random body-blow red herring that was this morning, I will not worry. I look forward to a time of future ignorance when, discharged, the bodies of my children will be closed, black-box systems whose inner workings are once again their own dark and clever business.

DAY FORTY-NINE

Friday, 20th November

As we inch closer to home an old, deep part of my soul has begun to stir and waken. Like Sophie, one day soon I will be faced with the quotidian dilemma, the irreconcilable schism of identity that is the working parent. My children's needs will be in direct opposition to my own. For these are the simple facts – I want to be with them, I need to be with them, but I also need and want and long to write.

While their lives hung in the balance, there was nothing else. I barely even saw myself renounce everything that was my own. One day I looked around and it had gone, and I realised I had cast it all off without a thought: work, family, friends, body, pride in my appearance, clarity and independence of thought. For months I've been a mind in hibernation. As they heal it becomes permissible to have my own requirements, though I don't yet know how many, or which ones. But in the unimaginable world outside this hospital I am a novelist, with a novel that was due to be delivered today. It is time to make a plan.

My agent, Zoë, offers to come to the hospital. It is so tempting. I grieve every moment spent away from my girls; I do not have minutes to spare for travelling. But Zoë is my precious portal to work, and thus, today, she feels a gatekeeper to a crumbling but venerable old neighbourhood in my own private self. I would like one day to be readmitted. Forget the pram in the hall. I do not want my agent to glimpse the incubators in the hall that must look, in this moment I feel certain, the most sombre enemy of good art. I suggest that we meet in a cafe.

Zoë cares about you, Gabe begins, *if she comes here, if you help her understand a little of what's been happening she can help you talk to your publishers, she can explain to them.* All of this makes objective sense and I am instantly furious with him for saying it.

You're totally wrong, I interrupt, urgently gesturing around the ward, as though I am superintending all of it, responsible for all those tens of babies in Special Care, out there beyond the glass. *If she sees any of this, she will think I do not have time to finish the book, she will feel too sorry for me, she will want to let me off the hook.* Gabe says nothing: to be let off the hook was precisely what he had been trying to suggest. But if Zoë never really knows about all this, if she does not see the two fragile babies for whom we will soon be entirely responsible, she may continue to believe I can finish a novel. And if someone out there believes it, it seems fractionally more possible that I can. I remember now: I used to be a writer. One day, I want be a writer again.

DAY FIFTY

Saturday, 21st November

Anton has been charged with giving me a blood test. Anton and I are friends again; in fact, it is fair to say I love him. Gabe has made his peace with my devotion to the doctors here; his daughters have been saved by a senior team of four men and three women and if his wife is slightly besotted with all of them then it is a small price to pay. I would give each and every person here a kidney, if they asked (except for Kitty the agency nurse, naked in her interest in the teeny-tiny dolly babies, snapping on gloves to make minute, needless adjustments, disturbing their precious, healing sleep. She will have to fend for herself).

Anton is finding this all very jolly, a friendly diversion from the high-stakes daily graft of torturing vulnerable infants for their own good. In my own professional life (longed-for, dreaded, murkily recalled), a bad day would be one on which the words would not come, or the wrong words came, or perhaps hours before a deadline I had unearthed a series of adverbs studded into what I'd thought a page of clean prose and they would all have to be cleared away, rocks impeding the progress of my plough. I know but still cannot quite force myself to imagine what a bad day at work would look like in this place.

Anyway. For Anton today is not a bad day at work. The reasons for my blood test are murky, having to do with a bug found on the girls' latest tests, yet another virus that has no symptoms or side effects. Someone somewhere – administrative, I think – is interested in knowing whether or not I passed it to the girls in pregnancy.

But I really don't think you did, Anton says, unsheathing an enormous needle and brandishing it in my direction. *You've almost certainly carried it since you were a baby too, so I feel confident that this exercise is of questionable to zero value.*

You know, he says, stabbing, *I haven't taken an adult blood test for ages. Your veins are so … bouncy.*

I am unable to resist. *Is it too soon to say at least you found one?*

With this I win a shocked laugh. *Too soon. Far, far too soon, thank you very much. Be nice to the man with the needle in your arm.*

Sorry. If it's any consolation this is genuinely the least painful blood test I've ever had. A+++ to you.

Yeah, yeah. Whatever. He presses a ball of cotton wool into the crook of my arm. *Hold that.*

I have my arm folded up, compressing my fingers upon this spot when Amelia bounds in. She leans over to hug me and sees Anton holding aloft what is, in neonatal terms, a blood sample the size of a swimming pool. She stops.

What have you done to my friend? To me she demands, *Are you our patient now? Do you need me to change your nappy? What is going on?*

It's for almost no reason at all, Anton tells her, writing in biro on the label. *Don't give it a thought.*

I look again at Amelia, trying to pinpoint what it is that's different. She is in jeans and a flowered jumper; I have never seen her in mufti before. *You seem full of beans?*

She is back, Amelia says simply. *She is back and everything again is good.* I notice the faded mint-green ends of her ponytail are now a bright and celebratory baby pink.

Anton smiles; I don't know if he knows what she is talking about – nurses and doctors do not seem to share intimate stories with one another very much. But our little glass pod is filled with goodwill, and two babies lie in witness between us, on the road to recovery. There is joy here, and I hope the girls can feel it. Anton's wedding is coming up. Amelia and Dawn are back together. What pops unexpectedly into my mind is a Kurt Vonnegut quote that hangs in my friend Naomi's loo: *I urge you to please notice when you are happy, and exclaim or murmur or think at some point, 'If this isn't nice I don't know what is.'*

White winter light pours into a room as warm as summer, and good people are here, doing hard work well, and with their ministrations, our own danger is passing. Maybe in the wider world of birth announcements and uneventful pregnancies our lot has not looked covetable. But I now know our great good fortune, in this place. We are the lucky ones and I am grateful. Contentment is rare and must be grasped and weighed in the hands, turned over and studied and logged. We may not be out of the woods but, for now, let the records show: I am happy.

DAY FIFTY-ONE

Sunday, 22nd November

I don't know where they get off with their eavesdropping, these meddling nurses. On ward round this morning it was as if Deepak had been paging through my diary: they've told him everything. He knew that Gabe's annual conference begins in Hong Kong on Tuesday, the most important three days of his working calendar; he somehow also knew that Gabe had a flight long-booked, and no intention of leaving us. After examining the girls he turned on Gabe.

What is all this about Hong Kong?

Gabe looked startled.

It is very important for your work, yes?

Yes, but—

Then you will go. Deepak gave a small, firm nod. *Yes. You will go, and we will all hold down the fort.* Both Amelia and Noor are here, which should have tipped us off that something fishy was afoot. No doubt one of them is the leak but with both here I can never know. Both wear expressions of carefree, whistling innocence. So that's that. The staff have ruled. Gabe is off to Hong Kong tomorrow evening and it will be just us girls, left to have pizza parties and braid each other's hair.

After Deepak left, Amelia told a worried-looking Gabe that I will be fine, and we all know Amelia is always right.

*

Today was Anton's last shift before his wedding; I didn't know. He clocked off while I was asleep – asleep! – in my pastel-coloured recliner, holding both girls. Falling asleep holding a newborn is one of those no-nos about which we are endlessly warned. All the leaflets say that it is basically inviting Sudden Infant Death Syndrome; apparently babies decide to expire the moment their exhausted mothers close their eyes on the sofa. So I decided this morning, in a rare act of defiance, to make the most of the saturation monitoring.

A wire still runs from one foot to a monitor, displaying to nearby Noor and Tracey that Raffaella and Celeste were sitting pretty at around 99 per cent and 98 per cent oxygen saturation, respectively. No suffocation on the nurses' watch – an alarm sounds if the girls hold their breath for even a fraction of a second. And so I wrapped my snoozing babies to my chest with a muslin like the world's best teddy bears, and fell into the most peaceful slumber I've had since my own babyhood. I missed my chance to give Anton a hug. While we three snored he crept in like a good fairy and left a handwritten note on a piece of printer paper:

It seems your time with us is coming to an end. It has been a pleasure to get to know you and your beautiful family.

Anton

I care deeply for these many people whose work I wish I'd never had to know; good, kind people whom I wish I'd never had to meet. It cannot be easy for the nurses and doctors either; what broad shoulders they must need, to bear our palpable ambivalence towards them. But look here, at this note; Anton's are more than broad enough.

DAY FIFTY-TWO

Monday, 23rd November

Gabe does not feel good about being away but it was important he went; conversations are taking place in Hong Kong that will shape his whole working year. Meanwhile, conversations are taking place that will shape our non-working year, too. We are planning to go home. I spent the morning interrogating Noor about baby circadian rhythms, about weaning and teething and tantrums and car seats, about how on earth I am meant to know how many layers a baby ought to be wearing at any given time. It is joyous, and entirely surreal even to be imagining such a future.

Once we are home she has forbidden me from aspirating their stomachs after a feed to find out what they've taken. *One day the tubes will come out and you'll have to live with the uncertainty like every other mother in the world. In any case, why'd you need to know how many mls they've had? You ain't going to be keeping notes.*

I averted my eyes. Keeping hospital-style feeding charts is precisely what I had planned to do, possibly for ever. *Celeste visited this evening with her husband. At 7.45 p.m. she ate 300g roast chicken, four roast potatoes and a disappointing quantity of broccoli.*

Noor's stories about her own three daughters make me delight that I have girls. *Of course,* she said cheerily, *you ain't never going to sleep again. Teenage daughters are as bad for sleep as newborns.* Her son sounds sweet and courtly; she thinks I should have a few of those, as well, just to even things out. At seven thirty when I was packing up to leave for handover she presented me with a box of six cupcakes like the ones from the World Prematurity Day tea party, but these are covered in beautiful fondant flowers instead of macabre disembodied baby toes. She commissioned them from her sister-in-law, on the occasion of Gabe's first night away. *Don't eat them all this evening*, she said. I drew myself up with as much dignity as I could muster. I would never do such a thing. I will keep two for breakfast.

DAY FIFTY-THREE

Tuesday, 24th November

There was a festival air on ward round today. I felt that we were cherished and petted this morning, that everyone was pleased with the little corporation of the three of us, coming along by leaps and bounds here, in our little corner office. *Daddy isn't going to recognise these giants*, someone said, leaning over Celeste with admiration and Celeste, wide awake, showed off the new clear blue of her eyes, which has been developing like a slow Polaroid, these last months. She gazed up unblinking. *I am a baby, now*, she seemed to reply, with a moue. *So what?*

I bask and preen in their reflected glory. How well they are doing! And here I am, steering the ship, determined that Gabe will be impressed on his return. At last weigh-in, yesterday, they were a positively elephantine 2.196kgs and 2.080kgs.

Today, two grand decisions are made. The last remaining wire, the oxygen saturation monitor, is to go, and instead Celeste and Raffaella will lie on apnoea mats that will sound an alarm if they stop breathing but will otherwise keep themselves to themselves. No more numbers. No more charts. No more beeping. The screens above them are falling dark. And – this is so petrifying that a little ribbon of terror constricts around my chest – when I lift them from their apnoea mats to hold them, there will be no monitoring at all. They will be entirely free-range babies, untethered. At liberty to roam up hill and down dale. The second advancement, slipped in while I was still reeling from the implications of the first, was that, while I am in the hospital, the girls will no longer be fed three-hourly but will be demand-fed instead. Were they ready? Everyone nodded in agreement. Was I ready? Nobody asked.

And just like that, no more expressing. No more schedules. Just the girls, in charge of their own destinies. Their NG tubes remain because they will need feeding when I am not here, and are likely to be exhausted by all this work. But while we are together we will just follow our instincts, as mothers and babies have done since mammals first suckled young. As they leave, everyone is beaming back at us. We have become a beautiful thing, the triad of mother and nursing babes.

*

What in God's name is going on around here? It is no exaggeration to say that I have been feeding, or trying to, for five hours, without a pause.

When ward round ended I scooped up Celeste, unable quite to fathom the wirelessness of her. I lifted her up, so we were nose to nose. I spun around 360 degrees and no cables caught around my legs, nor tugged at her feet. She is the difference between a landline and a mobile phone – she has been like those calls we made, years ago, the handset in one hand, the Bakelite rotary in the other, stepping over the cable and back again, occasionally ducking beneath them or halting abruptly and reversing, at the limit of the slack. The girls still have NG tubes but those are short and hang loose, not anchored to anything. Now they could, in theory, go anywhere. To Sainsbury's! To Wimbledon! On a grand tour of the Pyramids! They could take tea at the Ritz, or a box for *Le nozze di Figaro* at Covent Garden! They are independent women and can move freely, where they please.

I had only moments to appreciate this miracle because Celeste had not had a tube-feed and was rooting and frantic within moments of my holding her. She latched like a dream, sucked with gusto and while I admired her instinctive embrace of this new baby life, she fell deeply asleep. It had been about ninety seconds. Then Raffaella woke up, and we had an identical experience except that she was unconscious again before she'd even swallowed a mouthful. Since then first one and then the other have woken hungry and furious, fed for a minute or two or three, fallen asleep and then roused to repeat the routine, at ten-to-fifteen-minute intervals. Within the hour both of them were roaring with frustration, red-faced and windmilling with distress. They are still not very loud, nonetheless, their lamentations reverberate in this glass box like an echo chamber. By lunchtime we were in Act Three of a Greek tragedy.

Tracey, meanwhile, is conspicuous in her absence. Shortly after ward round she presented me with a giant foam doughnut, supposedly to enable tandem feeding. I am not naturally coordinated, and the word tandem makes me think of bicycles, thereby instantly arousing my suspicion. I cannot fathom how to breastfeed them both at once. How do you retrieve the second baby from across the room, when you are already anchored to the first? *If they could only hurry up and learn how to use their bloody neck muscles*, I think. *Or better yet, a knife and fork.*

Nonetheless, for the best part of five hours I have had this doughnut strapped around my waist like a security device. I look as if I am about to jump into a swimming pool. I feel as if I have jumped out of a plane. I have snatched up baby after baby, I have been racing back and forth to spin my teetering plates to no avail. While one is nodding off on the breast, the other is rousing, furious. As the day goes on they are hungrier and hungrier; more and more exhausted by their rage and frustration. I do not need to aspirate their stomachs to know that they have taken very little, because any minute now my breasts are going to explode, like something that Wile E. Coyote might purchase from Acme. Milk drips down my front. Earlier I discovered that Raffaella would consent to lie back open-mouthed on the doughnut and have milk dripped into her mouth, like a college student beneath a vodka luge, but would make no further effort. Still, she must have taken something by this painstaking method because when I tried to put her back in her cot to comfort a distraught Celeste, she vomited spectacularly, over everything. There was sick on all her bedding, soaked through all her layers of clothing, and needless to say, all over me. While I changed her I sang to Celeste, who was by this point steaming like a kettle. Then Celeste got in on the action by pooing over absolutely everything, and vomiting with the effort.

Everything in this room is on fire.

Traitorous Tracey pops her head round the door. *How you going?*

I am losing my mind, I say to her, very seriously. *I have lost my tiny mind, it has rolled somewhere like a walnut, like a marble, and I may never retrieve it.* As I say this, there is a brief moment of silence from the cots and, without pausing to explain myself, I elbow past her and dash to the loo. I sprint across Special Care like Roadrunner. When did my life become a Warner Bros. cartoon?

In the silence of the cubicle I hang my head. I'm ravenous, and I have never been so thirsty. I check my watch to discover that the three months that have passed since this morning's ward round were, in fact, only four hours. It is 2 p.m.

I am washing my hands in the bathroom when my phone rings.

Only me, says Tracey, horribly cheerful. *They're both at it again, you'd best come back.*

I sprint back, realising only as I am strapping on my rubber ring that I forgot even to sip from the tap.

Tracey has helped me into what should be a tandem feeding session, Raffaella on the left, Celeste on the right, but they are all talk and no trousers, these girls. Both babies are snoring, open mouthed, and I am stuck in a hard hospital chair, the babies balanced on a small foam semicircle, one held in place beneath each arm. The closest surface on which to set one down is the filthy hospital floor, which for a moment I consider, but even that is too far away. I am trapped. I semaphore wildly for Tracey but she is sitting on the desk at the nurses' station, chatting to Pam.

Tracey, I hiss, but either she doesn't hear me or she is keen to finish an anecdote. I consider a fancy manoeuvre to escape, but we haven't come this far only for me to dash out tiny brains by accident, on the floor of Special Care. Each time she walks past is like trying to catch the eye of the gliding waiter in a white-cloth restaurant; it is so tempting but I cannot, must not, shout. My life is passing.

It is now 4 p.m. and neither girl has had a wet nappy since the earlier explosions. They are slowly dehydrating. Also I could be using this precious synchronised sleeping to eat or at least to pump, just a bit, so that I am not engulfed by raging mastitis.

Tracey relents and comes back. *I'm stuck*, I tell her, pouting. *I've been stuck for ages.*

That's two babies for you, she says cheerfully. *I'm not coming home with you.*

I am going, I say, drawing myself up with as much dignity as I can muster, *to get some lunch.* Damp patches bloom on the front of my vest.

Have you not eaten? she chides. *It's five o'clock!* I resist the urge to scream, *What was I meant to eat in here, the hand soap?*

In Pastry Place, I gaze with uncharacteristic enthusiasm at the array, and choose a Cajun Chicken Bloomer, because it looks to have the most filling. I am reaching the front of the queue when the phone rings again.

They're up, says Tracey, *and very hungry. My goodness are they telling us all about it. You'd best come back.*

I hurl the sandwich back into the chiller cabinet and sprint up the stairs. At least I may find some release from this engorgement. I cannot wait for the main elevator, which moves through the hospital at the speed of tectonic plates. I am taking the stairs two at a time, holding my aching breasts like they are something apart from me that I must carry. I throw myself back into my chair, part my shirt with the button-popping force of Clark Kent becoming Superman and, restored to my arms, the girls drink nothing but fall deeply and instantly to sleep.

For the next hour everyone in this room is crying, some of us, I think to myself, more demurely than others. Raffaella is purple with rage; Celeste has been wailing and thrashing with such force that her hat has slipped down over her eyes, like a hostage. I sense that learning to multitask is key and so I weep efficiently and in dignified silence, and without a break in my efforts.

When I get home, I pump for almost an hour. The milk keeps coming; like the children, my body has been conditioned to the metronome routine of hospital life and has not enjoyed this deviation. In my absence the girls have been restored to their usual three-hourly tube feeds, because the hospital acknowledges that I cannot demand feed remotely (and no nurse, I think tartly, is going to race in and out at the whim of any tiny madam). When I phone at 2 a.m., both the girls have lost weight.

I shift to feel the duvet damp beneath my hands, and when I look at the clock I realise that I had been sitting here unmoving for eighty-five minutes and the bottles have been steadily overflowing, drip by drip. It is inevitable I will spill milk everywhere when I detach the pump, but it doesn't matter, because I am crying again anyway.

DAY FIFTY-FOUR

Wednesday, 25th November

We have never met for breakfast before, but Sophie and
Kemisha have called an emergency summit. WhatsApp has
become my Magic 8-Ball: I can ask our group anything, any
time, and an answer comes back, instant and authoritative.
But not without judgement, I discover. In the middle of last
night, I was deemed 'alarming'.

You've lost it, Sophie says, peering at the display of Pastry
Place baked goods before ordering something ostensibly
healthy, with bran and carrot shavings. *You're not allowed to
lose your marbles, it reflects poorly on the rest of us. We've*

assembled for caffeine and carbohydrate to tell you to stop being such a big baby.

I am behind Sophie in the queue, and Kemisha is at the back. She leans around me. *Soph, she hasn't even sat down yet.*

Yeah, I haven't sat down yet. This is the worst-staged intervention ever. Have you tried the raspberry and white chocolate Danish?

It's good, says Kemisha, at precisely the same moment that Sophie says, *It's disgustingly sweet.* I order one as an act of defiance, to show Sophie that she does not control me.

Sophie and I both cash in one of our free coffees. It is astonishing but despite our many previous visits together Kemisha hadn't realised that Pastry Place has a loyalty programme and now she is filled with outrage, busily calculating how many free drinks she's missed. While she's multiplying aloud I swipe my card so her cappuccino is free too, overjoyed that there is something in the universe about which I have been able to educate Kemisha. We retire to a table against the wall, and I return to the point in hand.

I promise you I'm not losing my marbles. I'm stating plain facts: I can't possibly have twins. There's been a terrible administrative mix-up, twins is one baby too many. Possibly two. I don't need an intervention; I just need you to help me find someone who wants one of my children before Friday. That looks foul, I add, needlessly, indicating Sophie's bran muffin.

It is foul, thank you for pointing it out. And before you go on, yes, I know it's probably got as much sugar as that white chocolate thing which I now obviously wish I'd ordered. Whatever, I will savour my sense of moral superiority. Anyway, listen. Because of yesterday's demand feeding shenanigans you were having a dark night of the soul—

I wasn't— I interrupt, but she interrupts back.

You were having a dark night of the soul, but we have not all come this far for you to collapse like a weakling at the final hurdle. You're rooming in tonight. Get it together.

Kemisha says, *Soph and I were just wondering, were you going to demand feed before all this? What was your plan before the girls came early?*

And just like that, her question is enough. I look from Kemisha to Sophie and feel relief like the slow passing of a raincloud.

I have grown so used to following doctors' orders that I have lost sight of my own locus of responsibility. But in our post-hospital future I will finally be free to care for my daughters as I choose. My friends are reminding me of the mother I might once have been, of the liberty with which we would all have made our choices, away from the constraints and supervision of hospital. Their words put right yesterday's wrongness not by acting as yet another external force, but by making audible my own inner voice. My friends are returning me to myself. Not for the first time I think how much clearer everything in my life would feel if it were decided by a committee of Sophie, Kemisha and me (I am willing, I think graciously, to take one third of the responsibility). But I know what they are trying to demonstrate this morning is the opposite. For better or worse, I am the one driving this bus.

Demand breastfeeding is not the natural conclusion of a hospital feeding programme. Demand breastfeeding is not a medical necessity. It is a social programme, and a hospital policy. It is merely a *suggestion*. It is, and I now see this with crystalline foresight, for me and for my family, the way that madness lies. I have exhausted premature twins, and demand breastfeeding does not suit them.

And – I throw back my shoulders at the unfamiliar subversive self-assertion of such a thought – it doesn't suit *me*. In our future life outside this hospital I too will once again have needs, and with this decision I shall accommodate them. One of my needs will be to stay sane. And so I will feed the children three-hourly, like the good, sweet little robot babies they have been trained to be.

Sophie has her head cocked to one side, observing me like a science experiment, watching the wheels turn. *The thing is,* she says, reading my mind, *I know everyone's all about demand feeding here, but that's a policy inherited from the labour ward, it doesn't necessarily suit premature babies, and in any case you have twins, so that's different, too. There has to be a bloody upside to this incarceration, and an established routine is surely one of them, for God's sake.*

I think about last week's session with a speech and language therapist, how the tip of her finger in Celeste's mouth for three sucks had so exhausted the baby that afterwards she had not had the strength to feed at all. I think of Raffaella, nursing doggedly for a whole fourteen minutes before her eyes rolled back in her head with full-body fatigue from which she barely stirred the rest of the day, sleeping through a nappy change, a repositioning, all her medications, several feeds. Aspiration showed she had taken precisely 2ml of milk in almost a quarter of an hour. They are a world away from having the strength to feed themselves. *I always planned on a routine, before,* I admit. And while we are blaspheming I venture, *Maybe I should try them on a bottle.*

Kemisha nods. *We were saying that, too. Otherwise, if you're waiting till they're both fully breastfed to get rid of the NG tubes it's going to be months.* As she says this I realise that it is true. They are not days but months away.

Sophie adds, *It just seems a shame to keep the tubes longer than you need when you can speed things up with a bottle. The flow's so much faster. Breast milk is breast milk. And demand feeding really seems mad for little twins. At the moment you have them calm and trained, reflux controlled, calorie intake where it should be, weight gaining, on a routine that is just about manageable for two parents who as it is will probably have to forego eighty to eighty-five per cent of their night-time sleep. Why not make life a tiny bit easier on everyone? And why not give Gabe the chance to keep feeding them, too, after all this?*

If yesterday was slapstick Warner Bros. then today has begun Disney sweet – cartoon bluebirds fly in heart formation above my head. *All right then,* I think, *three-hourly feeds it is. Three-hourly feeds I can do.* I will love and care for my children according to my own instincts, even if those instincts must be coaxed into life after a long-enforced hibernation beneath the snows of NICU. I have made a holistic decision for our family. It takes two mothers to remind me what it is that mothers do; what it is that mothers are.

Day Fifty-four

I say, *They'd shoot us all if they heard all this bottle talk.*

Oh, stop being such a wet blanket.

You are seriously into the tough love thing today, I grumble, but then I give Sophie the iced top of my pastry, the bit I have been saving, because she deserves it.

*

Nasogastric Competency Statement
For babies going home with NG Tubes

- I understand the importance of hand washing before and after feeding
- I have been shown how to correctly test the position of the feeding tube
- I know how to use the pH indicator strips
- I know which syringe to use to test the tube and which one to give the milk with
- I know how to attach the syringe to the feeding tube and remove the plunger to start the feed
- I understand that the milk must flow slowly and know that this is controlled by how high and low I hold the syringe

- If my baby vomits or changes colour or coughs, I know how to stop the feed quickly
- I know what to do with the syringes and bottle when the feeding is completed
- I know I must ask for help if I am unsure or worried about anything

*

There were beds here all along. Three private rooms at the very back of Special Care that resemble university dorms, with their beech-laminate furniture, fluorescent strip lights and sealed windows through which even the most determined could not see to throw themselves or, I suppose, a relentlessly wailing baby. There is a single hospital bed, a bedside table, a wardrobe and a lot of empty floor space into which my two children will soon be ceremonially wheeled, like tea trolleys at a conference. Here we must play house for a prescribed twelve hours under the side-eye supervision of the night staff, a rite of passage before discharge. I wonder if anyone ever fails, and what happens if they do.

Evening handover is finished and I am back in Special Care, in pyjamas. I cheated, and during my exile I raced home, had a shower, brushed my teeth, took out my contact lenses. Now I know the deal, I am taking no chances. I will not be leaving the bedroom under any circumstances, because earlier today, Noor told me that she's confiscating our apnoea mats. The babies will have to be just ... babies. Disconnected. Babies, Unplugged. It is enough to make me want to cancel the whole experiment: at the very least I should have waited for Gabe so we could take turns sitting up, to whisper words of semi-threatening encouragement like those parent-coaches at the Olympics: *In, out, yes, very good, now just keep doing that, well done, breathe in, now breathe out again ...* One or both of my children will almost certainly expire spon-taneously in the night, while I am two feet away sleeping the sleep of kings, in my fully-adjustable plastic hospital bed.

After this morning's Pastry Place intervention I have made my game plan. Overnight the girls will be entirely tube fed; Deepak wholeheartedly agreed when I said this on ward round earlier, though across the room I spotted the lactation-specialist giving the back of his head a filthy look. We will do our breastfeeding practice by day and by night they can rest, and recover for the following day's assault. Tube feeding means that they can rest. It also means that I cannot.

DAY FIFTY-FIVE

Thursday, 26th November

It is morning and I feel magnificent. I could, if called for, rule the world. I have changed ten nappies, and administered ten tube feeds, each of which takes in the region of six to fifteen minutes. Oh, and I did most of it attached to a hands-free double breast pump. Everyone is alive and I did not have to make use of my resuscitation training, which is good, because I have forgotten all except the part where you bellow *MY BABY ISN'T BREATHING* at passers-by. I feel an urge to run victory laps around Special Care. I may be just the tiniest bit hysterical. Noor, on again for the morning, eyes me with suspicion.

That's all fine, she says after I give her my blow-by-blow, obviously sorry to be the one to burst my bubble, *but when exactly did you sleep?*

I didn't, I trill, *I haven't slept one bit. I didn't even lie down! A few times I sat, for a bit, but then one of them would cry so I stood up again. They were both asleep at the same time for precisely no minutes at all.*

And your plan going forward is …?

Well, obviously, I tell her, jauntily kicking the brake off Raffaella's cot to help wheel the girls back out to their traditional station on the ward, *my plan is to go home and sleep right now, while you look after them.* I stamp the brake on, with emphasis. Then I grab my bag, meticulously packed since 4 a.m.

That ain't a sustainable plan, Noor calls after me, but her words are lost as I am racing through the lobby away from her as fast as I can. She, unlike me, is not allowed to leave the ward.

DAY FIFTY-SIX

Friday, 27th November

Gabe is back! He's back! He's in a cab, on his way home from Heathrow. He has to go home and scour off the swine flu and measles and flesh-eating bacteria to which I am convinced he has been exposed on the plane, but then he's coming to be trained up to my elevated medical standing. I am basically a neonatologist, now: before rooming in I watched a nine-minute resuscitation video and then this morning Amelia gave me a brief seminar on how to replace the NG tube when the girls yank it out, which in essence boils down to: don't stick it into a lung. Quite frankly, Gabe has a lot of catching up to do. But once he attains my expert standard that is it. We are free! Despite the feeding tubes, which will be temporary, the girls are cooked, almost ready to begin their careers as full-term, full-time newborns. The idea of walking out with them this afternoon feels both surreal and impossible, like shoplifting an expensive item from a department store: some hidden electronic tag will sound and security guards will descend on us, returning our stolen treasures to their rightful place on the ward. But Thomas says we can. Deepak isn't on today for us to say goodbye, but in any case we have an outpatient appointment with him in three days. No clean breaks, here. Like that hung-up ex-boyfriend who keeps wanting to meet up and hash things over, the hospital isn't going to let us walk away that easily. We will be back for audiology and ophthal-mology, dermatology and cardiology, for sessions on weaning and on motor development, and also to touch base with Deepak every twelve weeks, probably for years. Secretly I'm glad we will be popping back so soon; how much can I really fuck up between now and Monday?

The day proceeds as usual, except for two elephants in the room: a pair of car seats, kitted out with an extra padded insert for premature babies called a Tiny Traveller, bought from a specialist online boutique. They are, in fact, the grey of elephants, and look cosy, thick rolls of padding and Velcro to make our babies baby-sized. Tiny Travellers for our tiny travellers, though not so tiny now: on their discharge notes (already signed), their weights are 2.224kgs and 2.102kgs.

My parting from Amelia is a kiss blown through the glass; she is on admissions today and so is running past on soft rubber soles towards the labour ward. A new baby is on his way into the world, too early. Amelia will be part of the team there to greet him, to tend to him, to help him live. I want to tell his mother, *He could not be in better hands, nor meet a better soul, as his first encounter with humanity*. I know I will see Amelia soon. I will invite her and Dawn over for tea and plum cake. There is no plum cake big enough to contain my gratitude to Amelia. Still.

Then as always Sophie rescues me from myself, and from the buzzing mosquito of ambivalence that has been bothering me, in my nervous happiness. *Fuck you*, she texts, breaking the day's silence between us.

I know. You soon.

V. soon, we're rooming in next Tuesday. Day after Kemisha and Evanee. You've started an exodus.

Rooming in next week means both William and Evanee will be going home with oxygen support. Breathing alone is their final hurdle, as ours is feeding.

I'm such a trend-setter. So you're going for it?

Yup. Let's blow this hotdog stand, as a great woman once said. Think of the Michelle Obama arms I'll get, carrying those oxygen tanks around.

I think you're bloody brave.

I am, I'm quite excellent, thank you for noticing. I couldn't do NG tube at home, so right back atcha.

We are each least frightened of the thing we each must do. How clever nature is.

*

The car is at the door of the side exit – a light rain is falling. As Gabe and I run the babies to the car, one, two, a fine mist falls upon their faces, waking them. *Sorry, girls*, I whisper as they stir and stare, but then I begin to feel a tightening coil of disbelief. Sharp fresh air now, and rain, and low dark city sky above. But one day snow to taste and puddles for small wellingtons to stamp in, and the sensation of coarse sand pulled out beneath their feet by the recession of a wave. Ahead is teething and rolling and tasting and running; first bikes and goldfish funerals and big-girl beds, potty training and baking fairy cakes, standing on a chair to reach the kitchen table. Fights and hair-pulling and rows over bedtime; purées and dropped food and the endless wiping and re-wiping of highchairs; homework and missing puzzle pieces; birthday parties and swimming lessons; relentless winter colds. Nappies and nappies and nappies and nappies. One day I will know the sound of my daughters' laughter; I will hear their voices rise across the busy chatter of a playground, two ringing silver bells. One day in their cots they will lift their arms to me.

It comes upon me at once, in a rush, and my stomach falls away as if at the crest of a rollercoaster. I have been calm till now, I understand, because I did not allow myself to fantasise, nor to believe in my right even to imagine a future in which Gabe and I have two little girls, Raffaella and Celeste. Now I think, to envisage these things is not complacency, nor hubris. It is hope. I have walked our path with one foot in front of the other, gaze fixed upon the ground. Now, suddenly alert, I lift my head. It was all, all of it, awoken by this: the first sight of raindrops glistening on my daughters' brand-new eyelashes.

My children were born fifty-six days ago. Today, I am released into the world, a mother.

EPILOGUE

DAY ONE, AGAIN

Saturday, 28th November

In Dusseldorf, Germany, 117kg Tyson Fury (birth weight: 500g) beats 117kg Wladimir Klitschko, becoming Heavyweight Champion of the World.

We are home. My family is home.

Acknowledgements

I am grateful to Mishkenot Sha'ananim and the Marie Fellowship for the space and tranquillity and time to work, both in Jerusalem and in Venice. The British Library has been a refuge, as ever. For my magnificent agent, Zoë Waldie, Stephen Edwards and Laurence Laluyaux, my meticulous and dedicated editor Clara Farmer, Harriet Dobson, the wonderful Bethan Jones and Victoria Murray-Browne, and everyone at RCW, Chatto and Vintage, thank you. Thank you to Beth Coates, and Rachel Cugnoni. It is a privilege to have a home on such a list.

I owe a debt to my cherished, and frankly petrifying, first readers, for having the faith and generosity to bully me into writing the book in the first place, over kedgeree, last winter. You know who you are. Thank you also to Liz, for encouraging and inspiring, in this as in all else.

Thank you to Charlie Coleman and Adam Steingold, who read with intelligence and generosity. Thank you to Davinia Ferner-Robson, Jo Barlas, Caren Lerner, Bena Gershon, Nicola Avery-Gee, Boudien Moerman, Sophie Skarbek-Borowksa, Susannah Okret and Naomi Alderman for your wisdom and friendship. Thank you to Rupert Whitten for late night deliveries of Julia Donaldson and Haribo. Natalie Bellos applied her considerable brain and thus found this book its only possible title. Dr George Miller has been unstintingly generous with his medical advice from across the Atlantic, not only by reading this book but also while the children were in hospital. Thank you to my adopted godfather Dr Rodney Rivers, for reading this manuscript with such care, and catching medical omissions and errors. Any that remain are entirely my own.

I am grateful beyond measure to the National Health Service, and in particular to the nurses and doctors of the Central and Local Hospitals, whose individual praises I cannot sing out of respect for their professional privacy. Thank you not only for caring for our children, but also submitting to be written about with grace and good humour. Our special people, I do hope you know who you are. This book is a love letter to my husband, to my daughters, but it is also intended as a hymn of praise to the compassion, generosity and fundamental values of our National Health Service, and I hope it is thus felt. Long live the NHS.

I have striven for accuracy wherever possible but an exhaustive study of our time in hospital would have been impossible (not to mention unreadable) and several beloved people have been omitted from these pages. Katherine and her son Archie became as important as Sophie and Kemisha in the weeks and months after our discharge. We came to know one another only after its final page, still, their absence from this book feels wrong. Like Evanee, Archie was born at just twenty-four weeks, and the round of recent birthday celebrations for these babies was as full of disbelieving joy as you might expect. Lisa Wolfryd (who accidentally saw Gabe naked in the hospital bathroom) is now a treasured friend, despite having only a brief cameo here.

Out of respect for their privacy, our families appear here very little. Thank you to my mother, Karen, for unending emotional as well as gastronomic sustenance. My deepest love and gratitude go to my sister, Miranda, my best friend and favourite sidekick, whose kindness and generosity are an example to her nieces. Cathy Robson has always been my dream big sister, and her love and wisdom helped immeasurably. My mother-in-law Jenny saved us with the only hand cream that could counter the relentless anti-bacterial hand-washing (Norwegian Formula, for anyone who might need it) and both she and my father-in-law David delivered with great love innumerable barbecued lemon chickens, long after we were discharged.

For Gabe, quite simply, everything. I cannot begin to imagine what wonders I must have wrought in a former life to deserve you in this one. I am grateful every day.

And for my beloved Raffaella and Celeste, my funny, humbling, captivating beauties, every word of this book is a love song. You are our greatest gifts. Today is your third birthday, and you have already long-fulfilled our wildest dreams and made us proud beyond measure. You cannot know how we love you – thank you for fighting.

To the women of the milking shed I owe a debt that is all but impossible to quantify. Comradeship, wisdom and sanity lay in your hands. Sophie, Kemisha, Katherine, Lisa, Daniella, Jess, and many others who spoke casual words of kindness they may not even remember. And to the babies: William, Evanee, Archie, Emma, Phoenix. It is a privilege to watch you grow.

We are the lucky ones, and are humbled by it. This book is also for a brave little redhead, Raphael Charles Csemiczky, 4th October 2015 – 30th November 2015, *in memoriam*. Rafi's story isn't in these pages because it wasn't mine to tell. It was his, and is his family's. But Jess and Pete, we, the women of the milking shed, were privileged to know you right from the beginning as the devoted parents you have always been, long before the miracles of Ezra and Matilda. We knew Rafi and by your side we remember him, your beloved Ginger Ninja, our fallen soldier. זכרונו לברכה. May his memory be a blessing.

Francesca Segal
2nd October 2018

penguin.co.uk/vintage